Confidence In Full Bloom

A 30-Day Guide to Growing Unshakable Confidence

in Uncertain Times

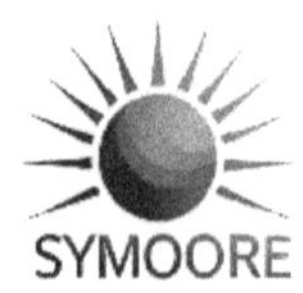

Published by
SYMOORE Publishing
ISBN: 978-1-961228-07-8

This

Confidence In Full Bloom

30-Day Guide to Growing Unshakable Confidence in Uncertain Times

was gifted with love and devotion to:

____

From: ________________________ on _______________

Welcome Beautiful Bloomer.

This is your space to grow unshakable confidence, even when life feels a little messy, uncertain, or overwhelming.

Imagine a bumblebee drifting from flower to flower across the cover of this guide: roses, sunflowers, dahlias, lavender, and mums, gathering energy, courage, strength, wisdom, and beauty from each bloom.

From that collected goodness, she builds a golden honeycomb: strong, sweet, and enduring.

That's you. Every small act of care, reflection, and courage is nectar for your growth, shaping your gifts into something precious you can savor and share.

Over the next thirty to ninety days, you'll plant seeds of self-worth, self-efficacy, and self-love. You'll water them with attention, intention, and courage, and watch your confidence rise, steady, bold, unstoppable.

Each practice, reflection, and ritual in these pages is a mirror, reminding you: your worth is real, your voice matters, and your power was never up for debate.

It's time to bloom.

Fully. Fiercely. Beautifully.

With love, light, and a wink of revolution,

xoxo,

Stacey

Contents

Prologue: Tea for Three at L'Air

The afternoon sun slipped through the courtyard trees at the Kimbell, scattering dapples of light across the white tablecloth I had ironed that morning. The air smelled faintly of jasmine and bronze, the kind of scent that only comes when metal, leaves, and history have spent decades in quiet conversation.

We were four women that day: Delicia, Rosie, Cara, and me, gathered for tea beside the sculpture *L'Air*. She reclined in all her bronze glory, a woman poised mid-float, suspended between earth and sky. Her form was both grounded and free, as if the weight of the world couldn't quite hold her down. I'd chosen this courtyard deliberately. I wanted my students to feel what freedom could look like; soft, luminous, unapologetically feminine.

It was graduation week, that strange season of endings and beginnings. Each of these women had reached a hard-won milestone during some of the most unpredictable years we've known, pandemic years, layoffs, family losses, global uncertainty. The kind of times that test your sense of worth until you almost forget you ever had any.

So instead of the usual classroom send-off, I told them, *"Come have tea with me."* A simple invitation, but I meant it like a blessing.

I'd brought the tablecloth from home, pressed so smooth it nearly shimmered. A small floral arrangement anchored the center, a mix of cream roses and lavender sprigs, cut from my garden that morning.

On each plate rested a linen napkin and a handwritten note tucked into a tiny gift bag. And because I believe confidence deserves a little ceremony, I handed each woman a fascinator hat when she arrived.

You should've seen their faces, surprise, delight, disbelief. Cara laughed, half protesting that she hadn't done her hair for a hat. Rosie blushed and tilted hers like she was channeling Lady Mary from *Downton Abbey.* And Delicia, who had shown up in my class months ago wearing hoodies like armor, just stared at her reflection in the teapot for a moment, then smiled.

That was enough for me.

The café staff had set out the tea stand, three tiers gleaming with little sandwiches, scones, and bright strawberries. The teapot itself, glass and silver, caught the afternoon light like amber honey. Steam curled up between us, and for a moment the whole world seemed to exhale.

We poured. We sipped. We breathed.

I told them how proud I was. How each of them had not only finished their studies but done it while holding down jobs, caring for families, pushing through self-doubt that could've stopped them cold. They'd done the hard thing. They'd made it here.

But when I said, "You must feel so proud," they each gave the same small shrug, the one women perfect somewhere between adolescence and adulthood. That practiced grace of deflecting praise.

Delicia spoke first, tracing the rim of her cup. "I thought I'd feel... something. You know? Accomplished. But mostly, I just feel tired."

Rosie nodded. "Same. Like I should be celebrating, but my brain's already saying, 'Okay, what's next?"

Cara sighed. "I can't even take a compliment without thinking I don't deserve it."

I sat back, the tea cooling in my cup. Their words weren't new to me, I'd heard versions of them from so many women before, but hearing them now, from these brilliant young women at the brink of everything, pierced something deep.

There we were, surrounded by art that had survived wars and centuries, sipping from porcelain, wearing little hats fit for duchesses, and still, inside, they questioned their right to be there.

It hit me: this wasn't just about confidence. It was about conditioning.

We'd been raised in a world that grooms women to shrink before they shine. To apologize before they speak. To measure their worth in approval, productivity, perfection, anything but self-love. Even at a table set for celebration, the ghost of "not enough" still finds a seat.

I looked up at *L'Air,* her bronze body stretched in mid-motion, unashamed and serene. Aristide Maillol had sculpted her as a monument to those lost in flight, but to me, she looked like every woman I've ever taught, rising, balancing, daring to believe she could float above the noise. Her skin, darkened by time, seemed to glisten with sunlight. She wasn't striving. She simply *was.*

"Look at her," I said softly, nodding toward the statue. "She's the reminder. You don't have to earn your right to exist in beauty."

Delicia turned, following my gaze. Rosie leaned in. Cara smiled faintly. For a few long seconds, no one spoke. We just watched her, this goddess of air, both strong and delicate, forever in the act of becoming.

I thought about all the tables women have been denied through history, the boardroom, the studio, the altar, the dinner party, the decision-making circle. But also, the quieter ones, the tables of affirmation, belonging, grace.

This tea was our reclamation.

We began to talk; not about grades or goals or what came next, but about belonging. Delicia shared how she'd grown up the only girl in a house full of brothers, always told to "toughen up." Rosie admitted she'd built a career around pleasing everyone but herself. Cara confessed that every success felt like a fluke, like she'd somehow fooled the world into overestimating her.

Their voices trembled, then steadied, like a string quartet finding harmony after a few uncertain notes.

I told them that confidence isn't loud. It's not the voice that announces itself. It's the whisper that says, *"You belong here."* And sometimes, that whisper needs witnesses.

That day, *we* were the witnesses.

We toasted to the small victories, the mornings they got out of bed when grief said stay under the covers, the nights they studied with babies sleeping on their laps, the days they showed up even when their hearts weren't sure.

We talked about *Bridgerton*, about Queen Charlotte's towering wigs and that quiet power in her eyes. About *The Gilded Age* and how women like Bertha Russell used the trappings of society to rewrite the rules. About *Downton Abbey,* where every cup of tea was a negotiation between duty and desire.

"See?" I said. "Every era has its table. Every woman has to decide how she'll take her seat."

By the time we finished the second pot, laughter had replaced the self-doubt. Delicia straightened her shoulders, adjusting her fascinator like a crown. Rosie leaned back, glowing. Cara reached for another scone and said, "Maybe I *am* proud of me."

Maybe she didn't even realize she'd said it. But we heard it.

And that's how confidence blooms, not in grand declarations, but in the small, honest confessions of *enoughness*.

Before they left, I handed each of them her gift bag. Inside: a journal, a small mirror, and a single line written in gold ink. "You are already the masterpiece. The world is just catching up."

We hugged in that glass courtyard, our reflections shimmering on the windows, *L'Air* behind us like a guardian spirit. For a fleeting moment, I swear she looked alive, the bronze breathing, her arms suspended not by gravity but by grace.

As they walked away, I thought about every woman who's ever doubted her worth, every one of us who's accomplished something and still asked, "Why don't I feel it?"

This book, this journey, is my answer. Because you, too, deserve a seat at this table.

The one where the tea is poured, the laughter flows, and the truth is spoken gently but clearly: You are not behind. You are not broken. You are blooming, right on time.

Blooming Reflection ; Why L'Air?

> When I first stood before L'Air in the Kimbell's courtyard, I didn't just see bronze, I saw becoming.
>
> Aristide Maillol designed her to honor a lost flight crew, but what I felt was something deeper: the eternal rise of women who keep lifting, even when the world tries to weigh them down. Her body, sculpted in motion, floats between earth and sky , strong but surrendered, powerful but at peace.
>
> That balance is what confidence feels like. Not perfection. Not arrogance. Just the steady grace of a woman who knows who she is becoming.
>
> I chose that courtyard for our tea because I wanted my students , and now you, to see that image reflected in themselves. You, too, have survived storms that no one saw. You've held your breath through the turbulence and still managed to land on your feet.
>
> L'Air reminds us that confidence isn't about standing taller than others; it's about remembering that we, too, can float.
>
> So, as you journey through these pages, imagine this: sunlight on bronze, tea in hand, laughter rising through the leaves.
>
> That's the energy you're stepping into. That's your air.

Introduction: A Seat Is Waiting for You

"Sometimes confidence begins not with a roar, but with the quiet clink of a teacup and the courage to sit down at the table."

The courtyard had grown quiet by evening, laughter still echoing faintly in the air. The chairs we'd pulled close sat slightly askew, as if remembering the women who had occupied them. The scent of lavender and lemon lingered, mingling with the faint metallic hum of L'Air.

I lingered too, reluctant to disturb the beauty that had bloomed between us. There was something sacred about that table. Not the tea or the flowers or the hats, but the space itself, the pause, the permission, the way stillness turns into strength when women feel seen.

As the light dimmed, I realized this wasn't just a celebration. It was a mirror, a reflection of how often women reach milestones without the joy they've earned, because the world taught us to achieve, not to believe.

So, I thought of you...

you, who keeps showing up, even when no one claps.

You, holding everything together; work, family, hope, while wondering when it will finally be your turn to rest.

You, smiling through exhaustion, editing yourself to fit the room, downplaying your brilliance because someone once told you confidence was arrogance, or that you were "too much."

You, standing at your own threshold, diploma in hand or heart in recovery, quietly asking, "Why don't I feel complete yet?"

You might not have been at the Tea For Three table, but a seat is waiting for you just the same.

The invitation is open, the cup is warm, and the conversation is real. This book is that table, your place to exhale, reflect, and remember who you are beneath the noise.

Because confidence doesn't always arrive polished and poised. Sometimes it shows up barefoot, a little late, still carrying the weight of survival. It isn't loud; it's the quiet decision to begin again, even when no one's watching.

We live in a world that celebrates productivity over peace, hustle over healing, and applause over authenticity. But real confidence isn't a performance. It's a homecoming. A return to love. A deep breath taken when you finally stop asking for permission to be yourself.

That afternoon, when I looked at L'Air, the bronze woman caught mid-rise, weightless yet grounded, I saw every woman who's ever doubted her worth. Each one of us learning to rise without apology, to float without fear, to live with the grace of air and the strength of earth.

You don't have to earn your right to this seat. You were born worthy of it.

So, pull up your chair. Let the world spin for a while without your help. Pour yourself a little grace. This is your space to rediscover what was never lost, your worth, your clarity, your calm.

The tea is still warm. The seat is waiting. Here is what's on the menu.

The Journey: 30 Days to Remember You

This isn't a makeover. It's a homecoming, a return to love.

It's for the twenty-something learning her worth, the forty-something reigniting her fire, and the sixty-something deciding she's not done yet. Over the next thirty days, we'll walk through three phases that build upon one another, gently and powerfully.

Days 1–10: Self-Worth / Emotional Wellness

We'll unlearn the lie that you must earn your place. You'll get honest about what you feel and where you lost yourself trying to meet impossible standards.

Days 11–20: Self-Efficacy / Physical Wellness & Goal Setting

You'll rebuild trust in yourself through small, sacred promises. You'll reclaim your body as an ally, not an adversary.

Days 21–30: Self-Love / Spiritual Wellness

You'll come home to your wholeness, not by "finding your light," but by remembering your power.

Real Talk: What This Book Won't Do

This isn't therapy (though therapy is holy.) It's not a miracle cure or a hashtag challenge. It won't tell you to "manifest abundance" while your bills say, "*Sis you need an income stream.*" It won't ask you to "just think positive" when the world is still uneven. And it definitely won't tell you to "hustle harder" when you're already running on fumes.

What This Book Will Do

It will remind you that your roots are strong and that the things buried deep within you can never be replaced. It will guide you back to the truth that you belong to yourself first, and that your power doesn't expire. It will help you build confidence that breathes, steady, lived-in, sustainable.

You were not made to shrink to fit smaller rooms.

You were made to expand, like L'Air, both grounded and free, reminding the world what grace in motion looks like.

So, Here's What I'm Asking

Give yourself thirty to ninety days, a season, not to become new, but to remember yourself as a whole. To build confidence that outlasts titles, timelines, and trends. To remember: you don't need permission to bloom.

Your confidence matters. Your bloom matters. And it's never too late to grow again.

Blooming Reflection: Why Your Seat Matters

> Every table tells a story.
>
> Some were built to exclude us, quietly, efficiently, with rules unspoken but understood.
>
> But when we set our own table, everything changes.
>
> A seat matters because it symbolizes belonging by choice, not permission.
>
> It's where truth is spoken softly, where laughter rewrites old narratives, where women gather to remember that power doesn't always roar, it often pours gently, like a tea kettle.
>
> The table you're sitting at now, these pages in your hands, is a continuation of that sacred afternoon at the L'Air tea party.
>
> You've been invited not just to read, but to rise.
>
> Your seat is ready.
>
> Your real love story begins now.

Getting Started With Confidence

Before you bloom, get grounded.

Here's your quick start:

1. Learn Why: Peek at A Crisis in Confidence to see how we got here. (optional)
2. Learn How: Get the quick tutorial on using this guide to rebuild, sustain, or reclaim confidence.
3. Know Your Words: Scan the Bloom Words, your power language for growth.
4. Gather Tools: Journal, pen, quiet space, a cup of calm — whatever helps you root in. See Appendix A for the full list.
5. Start Growing: One page, one practice, one moment at a time.

A Crisis of Confidence:
The Toll and the Turning Point

> If you're the kind of reader who just wants to dive in, you can skip ahead to the next chapter.
>
> But if you like to see the full landscape, the receipts, the realities, the why behind our weariness, stay with me.
>
> This chapter is our deep breath before rebuilding.

A scroll through social media says it all. People are scared, not just for their own futures, but for the future of the world. The headlines shout. The comment sections snarl. And the late-night doomscrolling? Endless.

We're living in an age that feels uncertain by design. The economy wobbles. Politics fracture. Grocery bills make us gasp. And the news plays on a loop of heartbreak. No wonder so many of us feel not just tired but depleted down to the spirit.

"Confidence doesn't crumble overnight
it erodes slowly under the weight of uncertainty."

Across ages, incomes, and identities, women are in the middle of what can only be called a crisis of confidence.

Here's how we know...

Confidence can feel personal, but its decline is measurable. The numbers tell the story our bodies already know.

- **17 %** of U.S. women feel *very confident* about the job market, compared with **23 %** of men (Bizwomen, 2025). It sounds small, but hesitation often costs opportunity.
- **52 %** of women worry about job security after DEI program cuts (Forbes, 2025). Even progress feels precarious.
- Women are more likely than men to delay promotions or job changes because of economic uncertainty (Bizwomen, 2025).
- A 2024 HP survey found that while women rate themselves higher in empathy and technical skill, they remain *"over-mentored and under-sponsored."* Harvard Business Review and NIH studies confirm men still receive more powerful advocacy, keeping women stalled at leadership's threshold.
- Globally, women make up **41 %** of the workforce but hold just **29 %** of top management roles, and progress is slowing (World Economic Forum, 2025).

Beyond the Workplace

The confidence gap doesn't clock out at 5 p.m.; it follows us home, into our finances, our families, and our mirrors.

- Only **28 %** of women feel comfortable making investment decisions, compared with **39 %** of men; **58 %** say investing feels intimidating (Motley Fool, 2025).
- In STEM, **57 %** of girls uninterested in science careers say they "wouldn't be good at it," compared with **38 %** of boys

(Gallup/Walton Family Foundation, 2023). That's not a talent gap; it's a confidence gap.

- Among Gen Z women, those describing themselves as *thriving* dropped from **46 %** in 2024 to **37 %** in 2025, while men's numbers held steady (Gallup, 2025).

These figures matter, but they're only one window into a larger story.

The Bigger Picture

The same forces that chip away at confidence in the office; bias, precarity, unrealistic expectations, also shape how women see themselves at home, online, and in their own skin. When systems reward silence, when safety feels uncertain, when autonomy erodes one policy at a time, confidence starts to feel like a privilege instead of a birthright.

Women everywhere , working, caregiving, creating, surviving, are being conditioned to question their worth in a world that profits from their doubt. Even those with wealth or influence aren't immune; comfort only delays the reckoning.

Because here's the deeper truth:

The crisis of confidence isn't about careers. It's about control, belonging, and belief.

And this is where our work begins, the turning point where we decide to rebuild. Not by striving harder, but by remembering who we were before the world taught us to doubt it.

From Crisis to Impact

When confidence begins to crack, the mind feels it first, but the body always follows.

Every time you've swallowed words to keep the peace, smiled when you wanted to cry, or kept pushing through the ache because rest felt like weakness, your body kept the score.

It remembered every apology that wasn't yours to make, every meeting where you made yourself smaller, every night you convinced yourself exhaustion was "just life."

The truth is that confidence doesn't only live in your head. It lives in your heartbeat, your breath, your posture, your tone. It shapes how you move through the world, how deeply you sleep, how freely you laugh, how much space you allow yourself to take.

So, before we start rebuilding it, we have to understand what the lack of it has done to us. Because the toll isn't just emotional, it's physical, spiritual, and cellular.

Let's talk about that weight you've been carrying, the one no one else can see but you feel every day.

We'll do that in the next chapter, The Impact on Your Well-Being; The Invisible Weight Women Carry.

The Impact on Your Well-Being

THE INVISIBLE WEIGHT WOMEN CARRY

> If you're short on time, here's the short version:
>
> Confidence doesn't just shape how you feel; it shapes how you function.
>
> When self-doubt becomes chronic, it doesn't stop at your thoughts. It seeps into your body, your relationships, your spirit.
>
> This chapter connects the dots between emotional exhaustion, physical symptoms, and the quiet epidemic of women holding everything together while falling apart inside.
>
> If you're ready to dive straight into the work, skip ahead to the Key Concepts section.
>
> But if you've ever felt that bone-deep fatigue, or whispered, "Why am I always the strong one?" this part is for you.

The Real Weight

Let's stay in *real mode* for a minute, it's not just your imagination. The world does feel heavier than it used to. As I pointed out earlier, scroll any feed and it's all there: friends unraveling under pressure, coworkers chasing impossible standards, mothers juggling burnout like it's an Olympic sport. Even our *self-care* comes with a to-do list.

Women are holding up entire families, classrooms, companies, and communities, while quietly cracking in the corners.

We're laughing on the outside, crying in the car, and calling it resilience.

But here's another little shot of truth: when confidence wavers, it doesn't stay neatly in your head. It travels through you. It lives in your shoulders, your stomach, your sleep, your smile.

It sounds like this:

- Sleepless nights spent replaying what you *should've said.*
- Headaches that start as tension and end as migraines.
- A stomach that twists every time you have to speak up.
- A fatigue that no vitamin or vacation seems to touch.

These aren't random symptoms. They're the fingerprints of over-functioning, of being everything to everyone until there's almost nothing left for you.

Maya's Silent Stress

Maya was a mid-level manager who never applied for the director role she was more than qualified for. She told herself she "wasn't ready."

Behind the scenes, she worked ten-hour days, slept in fragments, and woke at 3 a.m. with her heart pounding. When her doctor diagnosed hypertension at thirty-seven, it wasn't just a medical issue, it was emotional overload.

Maya didn't have a blood pressure problem. She had a confidence problem.

Research backs her up: women with low self-confidence are significantly more likely to experience stress-related illnesses, migraines, insomnia, autoimmune flare-ups. The body keeps the score when self-doubt becomes a lifestyle.

The Whole-Self Impact

Low confidence ripples through every dimension of wellness:

Mind: It fuels anxiety, depression, and self-silencing, those quiet moments where you swallow truth to keep the peace.

Body: It keeps your nervous system on high alert. Tight shoulders. Clenched jaw. Racing heart. Skipped meals. Over time, that constant tension wears you down.

Spirit: It erodes joy. You forget the sound of your own laugh. You stop believing in what once lit you up.

"When confidence cracks, the foundation trembles."

Erica's Relationship Pattern

On paper, Erica seemed self-assured; career steady, style impeccable, but in love, she moved like someone waiting to be picked.

She'd never been taught that choosing was her right.

So, she accepted what arrived, mistaking attention for affection and persistence for love.

The men she dated praised her strength but chipped away at her peace.

One called her "too sensitive" when she asked for kindness.

Another disappeared for days, then returned with apologies she felt obligated to accept.

Each time, she quieted her intuition and told herself she was "understanding."

Like so many of us, Erica learned early that being wanted was safer than wanting too much. That love meant staying, accepting, absorbing.

Studies show that women with low self-esteem are more likely to tolerate mistreatment or remain in relationships that diminish them, not from weakness, but from conditioning.

We've been taught that endurance is virtue, that shrinking is safety, and that being chosen is the same as being loved.

Sophia's Scroll

Sophia, a college sophomore, spent hours comparing her life to digital highlight reels. Every scroll whispered, You're behind. Every unreturned like echoed, You're not enough.

Within months, she was skipping meals and calling it discipline.

What she didn't know was that social-media-driven self-comparison is now one of the leading risk factors for anxiety and disordered eating among young women worldwide.

We were raised on filters, digital and emotional. But no filter can hide the ache of self-doubt.

THE WELLNESS WAY FORWARD

The good news? Confidence can be grown. It is not fixed, and it is never too late. When confidence strengthens:

- **The mind** finds peace instead of panic.
- **The body** begins to heal as stress hormones settle.
- **The spirit** reconnects with purpose and joy.

That's what Confidence in Full Bloom is all about. It's not about becoming someone new, it's about reclaiming who you already are, and giving yourself permission to rise, to root, and to bloom.

Confidence is medicine for the whole self. And it may just be the most important health practice a woman can cultivate.

WHY THIS BOOK NOW?

Because we can't heal what we won't name. And we've been naming everything but the real wound, our depletion of confidence, our loss of ease, our quiet forgetting of worth.

Exhaustion is just how the body says, "I can't carry this much doubt anymore."

Confidence isn't a luxury; it's a lifeline.

It's what allows a teacher to keep smiling through chaos, a nurse to stay compassionate through fatigue, a mother to rebuild after loss.

It's what fuels women everywhere; from boardrooms to classrooms to kitchen tables.

And yes, the world is uncertain, volatile, messy, loud. But your confidence doesn't have to be. You deserve to walk into any room and know you belong there.

You deserve a voice that doesn't tremble with apology.

You deserve a peace that isn't swayed by headlines, hashtags, or anyone else's definition of your worth.

This book is here to help you rebuild your confidence from the inside out. Not the kind that begs for applause, but the kind that grows quietly; like deep roots remembering how to bloom again.

So, take a breath.

This is your season.

You've seen how confidence touches every part of your well-being, mind, body, and spirit. Now it's time to understand how it grows. Before we plant new seeds, let's get familiar with the soil.

In the next section, we'll explore the three roots of confidence: self-worth, self-efficacy, and self-love.

Now, let's take a look at some of the key terms and concepts that will help you bloom.

Confidence In Full Bloom Key Concepts

As you journey through this book you will realize that it is more than just inspiration; it is a set of confidence building Bloomprints for transformation.

Here are the key terms you need to know to when you read your bloomprints.

Bloomprint

> **Bloomprint (n.):** Your Bloomprint is the personal roadmap you follow to grow into your fullest self. Like a blueprint for a house, it gives structure and direction, but instead of walls and floors, you're building habits, mindsets, and moments of self-care.

Across the three phases of this journey, you'll follow a unique Bloomprint for each: Self-Worth (GROUND), Self-Efficacy (GROW), and Self-Love (BLOOM). Each one guides you with intentional practices designed to nurture your mind, body, and spirit in ways that are specific to that phase.

Each day, you'll move through a consistent rhythm:

- Morning – Begin with a mantra and reflection to set your energy and intention.
- Midday – Pause to reset with a grounding practice or empowering reminder.

- Bedtime – Close the day with reflection and gratitude, sealing in the growth.

Over time, this simple, daily pattern becomes a lifestyle shift. Your Bloomprints help you stack new, life-affirming habits, one on top of the other, until you've designed a life that feels rooted, radiant, and resilient.

Let's look at a few definitions that may come in handy as you bloom forward.

THE PILLARS OF SELF - CONFIDENCE

Just as flowers grow in stages, you, too, will unfold your confidence, layer by layer, into your fullest expression of self. This Bloomprint guides you through three essential nutrients that grow lasting confidence: self-worth, self-efficacy, and self-love, while tending the soil of self-esteem that holds it all together. Let's unpack each one so you understand how they work together to help you bloom.

Self-Esteem

> **Self-Esteem (n.):** Self-esteem is how you *see* and *feel* about yourself day to day; it's your personal evaluation of your abilities, qualities, and value. Think of it as the weather system of your inner garden. Some days, the sun is shining, you feel capable, confident, and ready to grow through challenges. Other days, clouds roll in and it feels harder, like blooming in a drought. A woman with self-esteem thinks: "I am worthy and enough just as I am.

Where does it come from? Self-esteem begins forming in childhood, shaped by the voices and experiences around us. Did people celebrate our efforts or only our successes? Were we loved unconditionally, or only when we were "good"? Did we feel free to be ourselves, or were we compared to others? Over time, these messages became the soundtrack we play back to ourselves.

How is it lost? Through life's pests and weeds: criticism, rejection, betrayal, toxic relationships, trauma, and the relentless chatter of our inner critic. Each sting chips away at our sense of worth, capability and belonging.

The good news: Self-esteem isn't fixed. It can be replanted, nourished, and strengthened, no matter how neglected or storm-tossed it has been. That's exactly what this book offers: a Bloomprint with practices, reflections, and at-home wellness therapies to help make changing your inner weather grow sunnier, steadier, and more resilient easier and totally doable.

Self-Worth

> **Self-worth (n.):** Self-worth is your belief that you are valuable simply because you exist. Not because of your job title, your relationship status, your weight, or your productivity levels. You are valuable because you are here, breathing, being, becoming.

When you strengthen self-worth, you stop negotiating your value with the world. You begin to honor your boundaries, make choices that align with your truth, and accept love not as something to be earned but as something you naturally deserve. Self-worth allows you to stand tall even when the world tries to shrink you, and to rest in your own skin without apology.

Where it gets lost: When we measure ourselves against impossible standards, tie our worth to other people's approval, or compare our behind-the-scenes struggles to someone else's highlight reel. When rejection or failure convinces us that we are less-than. When the noise of the world drowns out the truth of our inherent value.

Self-Efficacy

> **Self-efficacy (n.)** : Self-efficacy is your belief in your ability to handle life, get things done and reach your goals. It's the quiet but steady voice that says, "*I can handle this," or* "I can figure this out."

When you strengthen self-efficacy, you begin to trust your own choices and follow through on them, whether that's setting goals, solving problems, learning new skills, or bouncing back from challenges.

Where it gets lost: When life knocks us down too many times without a break. When we fail, and instead of seeing it as growth, we start believing we "can't." When others swoop in to rescue us so often that we stop trusting ourselves to rise. When things change so quickly, we feel like we can't keep up.

Self-Love

> **Self-love (n.):** Self-love is treating yourself with the same kindness, compassion, and respect that you give to people you adore. It's how you care for your own body, mind, and spirit, choosing rest, nourishment, joy, and forgiveness instead of neglect or punishment. It's how you speak to yourself, and how you prioritize your needs without guilt.

When you strengthen self-love, you become your own safe place. You create rituals of care that sustain you, from savoring a cup of tea to setting aside time for creativity or rest. You begin to replace self-criticism with encouragement, and punishment with patience. Self-love isn't selfish, it's soil. It's the fertile ground where your confidence takes root and where all other forms of growth become possible.

Where it gets lost: When we're taught to put everyone else first. When guilt or shame drives our choices. When we confuse self-sacrifice for strength or believe that our needs make us a burden. When old wounds tell us we are undeserving of our own kindness.

Self-Confidence

> **Self-Confidence (n.)** : Self-confidence is your steady trust in who you are, what you can do, and what you're worth. It's that calm, grounded assurance that says, "I've got this, even if I'm still figuring it out."

Real self-confidence isn't loud or flawless. It's the quiet harmony between your **self-worth** (knowing you're valuable), your **self-efficacy** (believing you can act and adapt), and your **self-love** (treating yourself with care, even when you fall short).

When your confidence is strong, you stop performing for approval and start living from truth. You speak up. You go after what matters. You bounce back faster because your worth isn't up for debate, it's a given.

Where it gets lost: Confidence slips when we grow up comparing, performing, or trying to earn love that should've been unconditional. It fades when failure or rejection make us question our enoughness, or when we spend so long proving ourselves that we forget to nurture ourselves. Those moments chip away at the bridge between who we are and who we believe we can be.

Self-confidence blooms back when self-worth reminds you that you deserve the good, self-efficacy whispers that you can make it happen, and self-love anchors you in the truth that you are already enough.

So basically...

Self-worth says: I matter.

Self-efficacy says: I can.

Self-love says: I will treat myself kindly while I grow.

Together, they form the foundation of steady, resilient self-esteem, the kind that blossoms into true confidence.

This book is your space to let that confidence, peace, and joy flourish; it's your seat at the tea table, resting in the graceful shadow of L'Air.

How To Use This Guide

Here is the skinny on your 30-day-ish journey to grow unshakable confidence , the kind that doesn't crumble when life gets chaotic. Notice that little "-ish"? That's because confidence, like healing, doesn't follow a perfect timeline. You'll grow one touchpoint at a time, one breath at a time, one small act of self-trust at a time.

Think of this book as your confidence companion , part coach, part calm voice, part mirror reminding you who you are. I'll meet you exactly where you are, and together we'll walk toward where you're meant to be grounded, capable, and blooming in your own power.

And yes , we'll keep it real, we'll keep it doable, and sometimes, we'll even laugh.

PRE-BLOOMING: Set Your Foundation (Do this before Day 1)

Before you dive into your 30-day practice, you need to prep your inner garden space for growth. You're not just learning *about* confidence , you're building it, nurturing it, and tending it like something sacred. You will find a list of tools in Appendix A.

1. Gather Your Tools & Claim Your Space

Grab your *Confidence In Full Bloom Journal* or one that speaks to your style. Create a cozy nook , a spot that whispers, *"This time is mine."* Add a candle, a cup of tea, maybe a little background music. You're signaling to your brain: this is my sanctuary. See the complete list of suggested Bloom Tools in Appendix A.

2. Take Your Pre-Bloom Confidence Quick Assessments

Each section has its own starting assessment. These aren't a tests; they are a reflection. You'll check in with where you're starting in each section , your stress levels, energy, and confidence baseline. Later, you'll take the same check-ins and actually *see* your growth, because confidence builds quietly and sometimes you don't notice it until you look back.

3. Build Your BYO Bloom Plans

Before each phase of your journey, you will have the opportunity to create your own menu of mini Bloom At-Home wellness practices, the little things that make you feel centered and alive. You may choose things like herbal tea blends, ancient stretching rituals, prayer, journaling, aromatherapy, playlists, meditation, whatever feels like nourishment. Confidence grows best in the soil of self-care. You will find a wonderful set of curated Bloom At-Home Wellness practices for each section that you can choose from in Appendix B. Feel free to add your own. Don't flake on this part of the journey. I repeat, DON'T Flake. You deserve this and you are the only person who can provide it for yourself.

YOUR BLOOMPRINTS: 30-Day Confidence Flow Segments

Confidence doesn't grow overnight; it unfolds in phases. You'll journey through **three stages**, each one building on the last:

- Phase 1: Self-Worth (GROUND) Believing that you are valuable simply because you exist.
- Phase 2: Self-Efficacy (GROW) Trusting that you can set goals, take action, and handle life as it comes.

- Phase 3: Self-Love (BLOOM) Treating yourself with compassion, care, and respect , the way you would someone you deeply cherish.

Each phase lasts ten days, but these aren't deadlines. They're invitations. Take your time, repeat what resonates, and let the lessons root deeply and authentically.

YOUR DAILY BLOOMPRINT RHYTHMS

Confidence loves consistency. Each day gives you three simple touchpoints , your anchors for staying grounded, centered, and connected to yourself. Here's what they might look like, based on the phase you are working through.

Self-Worth - Morning: GROUND + INTEND (10–15 min)

Set the tone for your day. Use your Bloom Essentials Breathe. Sip. Stretch. Speak a simple truth: *"I belong here."*

Self- Efficacy - Midday: GROW (10–15 min)

Use your preferred Bloom Boosters to help you pause with purpose. Do the daily practice , a reflection prompt, breathwork, or a small confidence stretch.

Self-Love - Evening: BLOOM + REST (10–20 min)

Unwind with gratitude and self-care. Acknowledge what went well. Let your body and mind rest in your own approval.

You're not adding more to your to-do list , you're creating touchpoints of wellness that recharge you instead of draining you.

MAKING THE MOST OF THIS JOURNEY

- **Go at your pace.** If you miss a day or need more time, take it. Confidence isn't a race; it's a rhythm.
- **Progress looks like practice.** Some days you'll feel unstoppable; other days you'll question everything. Both are part of growing.
- **Celebrate the small wins.** Every boundary held, every truth spoken, every moment you choose rest over pressure , that's confidence in bloom.
- **Stay connected.** Talk with trusted friends or your community as you go. Confidence may be personal, but it's also relational , we grow braver together.
- **Stay kind.** This work may stir things up , old doubts, buried fears, forgotten dreams. That's normal. Kindness is how you keep blooming through it.

At the end of the day, this guide is your permission slip to stop shrinking and start shining. The world doesn't need a more polished you , it needs a more present, powerful you.

Before you begin, take a moment to remember, growth isn't just something you plan; it's something you practice.

To make that practice tangible, I invite you to grow something alongside your blooming journey.

Because when you nurture life, when you water, tend, and watch something unfold, it mirrors the quiet transformation happening in you.

Grow While You Bloom

One of the sweetest ways to deepen your Confidence In Full Bloom journey is to literally grow something alongside it. Just as you're planting seeds of wellness, clarity, and joy within yourself, you can nurture a little plant that thrives as you do. Each new sprout and leaf becomes a gentle reminder of your own growth.

Try this:

Plant herbs or flower seeds in a small pot and place it somewhere you'll see every day, maybe near your practice space, by a sunny window, or even on your desk. Each time you water it, take a breath, and remember you're watering your own roots, too.

Easy-to-grow indoor friends include:

- Basil – fragrant, uplifting, and perfect for teas or meals.
- Mint – refreshing, great for digestion, and lovely in water or tea.
- Rosemary – grounding, aromatic, and a natural energy booster.
- Lavender – soothing scent, beautiful blossoms, and calming energy.
- Geraniums – cheerful pops of color that brighten your space.
- Spider Plant – nearly indestructible and an air-purifying champion.

Are you ready to get started? Let's get you going with Phase 1.

Phase 1:

Blooming Self-Worth

Your Self-Worth journey is officially underway. This first phase invites you to lay a strong foundation by honoring your inherent worth and nurturing your emotional wellness.

"When you know your worth,
you stop negotiating your peace."

Anchor List for Phase 1

1. Take Your Self-Worth & Emotional Wellness Assessments - Awareness is the first act of confidence

2. Create Your BYO Bloom-At-Home Wellness Plan- Choose rituals and rhythms that help you feel grounded and nourished each day

3. Meet Kyla - Your Phase 1 story companion.

4. Practice Self-Worth.

Blooming Self-Worth Quick Assessments

SELF-WORTH ASSESSMENT

Instructions: For each statement, rate yourself from **1 (Not at all true)** to **5 (Completely true).** Total your points at the end.

Part 1: Inner Beliefs

		1-5
1	I feel proud of who I am becoming.	
2	I believe in my own value and worth.	
3	I feel confident expressing my true self.	

Part 2: Daily Habits

		1-5
4	I take daily actions that uplift my mood or energy.	
5	I celebrate small wins in my life.	
6	I practice gratitude regularly.	

Part 3: Relationships & Joy

		1-5
7	I feel supported and connected to others.	
8	I notice and embrace joy in my daily life.	
9	I speak my truth with honesty and compassion.	

Total

See the Self-Worth assessment key on the next page. Then, complete the Emotional Wellness Check and set a goal for the next 10 days.

Blooming Self-Worth Quick Assessment - Scoring

- 9 –18: Your self-worth garden is ready for planting. This 10-day journey will help you nurture new roots of confidence.
- 19 – 31: You have some blooming buds of self-worth. During the 10 days, you'll strengthen and water them.
- 32 – 45**:** You already radiate a strong sense of self-worth. Use this journey to deepen and sustain your flourishing.

EMOTIONAL WELLNESS CHECK AND GOAL SETTING

This visual exercise helps you assess your current emotional wellness and set intentions for growth during Phase 1. You'll return to this same exercise on Day 10 to see your progress.

What This Measures

Your emotional wellness pie represents how well you're managing your emotional life right now. Consider:

- How easily you bounce back from disappointments
- Your ability to express feelings in healthy ways
- How much emotional energy you have for daily life
- Your capacity to comfort yourself when hurt
- How well you handle everyday frustrations

Instructions

Step 1: Measure Your Current Wellness: Look at the pie chart divided into four quarters (each worth 25% for a total of 100%). Using a colored pencil, crayon, or marker, shade in the amount that represents your emotional wellness TODAY.

My current state:

Shading Guide:

- **4 full quarters (100%):** You feel emotionally strong and resilient
- **3 full quarters (75%):** You feel mostly strong with minor challenges
- **2 full quarters (50%):** You feel balanced but could use improvement
- **1 full quarter (25%):** You feel this area needs significant attention
- **No shading (0%):** This feels very challenging right now. Perhaps I need to check in with a professional.

- **Partial quarters:** You can shade portions of quarters for more precise percentages. **Example:** If you feel your emotional wellness is at about 62%, you will completely shade 2 quarters (50%) and shade half of a third quarter (12%).

Step 2: Name Your Current State: On the line above your shaded pie, write a name that captures how you feel emotionally right now.

Examples of naming:

- "Emotionally Drained but Hopeful"
- "Frustrated but Functioning"

- "Fragile but Fighting"
- "Steady but Guarded"

Step 3: Explain Current State: Next to your pie, write 2-3 sentences describing:

- **Points of joy:** What's going well emotionally? Where do you feel strength?
- **Points of pain:** What emotional challenges are you facing? What feels hard?

Example: *"I've been acknowledging my wins more and catching those old 'I'm not good enough' thoughts before they spiral (growth), but I still find myself shrinking back when someone questions my ideas or overlooks my contributions (pain)."*

Step 4: Set Your 10-Day Goal

In the space provided, shade a second pie showing where you hope your emotional wellness will be after completing your Self-Worth development work. This becomes your target for the next ten days.

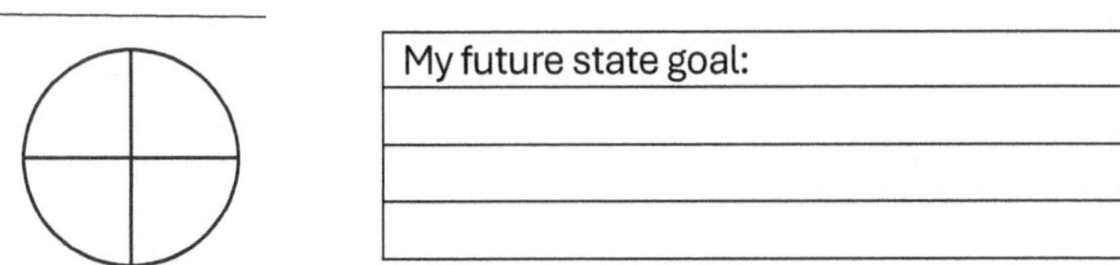

Goal-Setting Tips:

- Be realistic, aim for improvement, not perfection
- Focus on building skills rather than eliminating all emotional challenges

BYO Bloom At-Home Emotional Wellness Plan

This is your moment to design a wellness plan that speaks to your soul. See Appendices B: 1a and B:1b. Choose the Bloom At-Home Wellness practices that call to you. What helps you feel grounded, peaceful, safe, and whole? There's no right or wrong. Let your heart and health lead you. Use the space below to build you plan:

Plan 1

Sunrise	
Midday	
Bedtime	

Plan 2

Sunrise	
Midday	
Bedtime	

Plan 3

Sunrise	
Midday	
Bedtime	

KYLA'S STORY: RECLAIMING SELF-WORTH

Kyla was a sixth-year teacher who loved her students fiercely. She thrived on their laughter, their curiosity, and the small victories that filled her classroom with light. But after COVID, everything shifted. She felt the pull to return to in-person teaching before she thought it was safe. Living with her two children and her aging mother, who had diabetes, meant that every sneeze, every cough, and every crowded hallway carried stakes far beyond herself. Yet the mandate came down: return to the classroom or risk her career.

For weeks, she wavered between guilt, fear, and frustration. How could she keep her family safe while staying true to her students? How could she honor her own needs when every adult around her seemed to have an opinion about what was "right"? Kyla felt herself shrinking under the pressure, doubting her decisions and even her own worth.

The stress didn't stay in her head. Sleepless nights became her new normal. Her shoulders ached, her mind raced, and she carried a heaviness that felt permanent. Yet, amidst the exhaustion, Kyla realized something crucial: she had not lost her worth. She had simply lost sight of it under layers of obligation and fear.

Slowly, she began to reclaim herself, starting with small, intentional rituals.

Morning: Kyla lit a candle in her kitchen before the day began and brewed a calming cup of herbal tea. The rising steam and warm scent were tiny reminders that she mattered.

Midday: When the day threatened to pull her under, she took five minutes to step outside, breathe deeply, and reconnect to the body that had carried her family and students through so much. A short stretch or a walk around the playground became her act of self-respect.

Evening: Once her children were settled and her mother resting, she sank into the quiet with soft music, journaling reflections, and a gentle affirmation: *"I am enough. I am worthy. I matter."*

Over time, these small acts of care grew into something bigger. Kyla joined a local meditation group and discovered the power of shared stillness. She tried yoga flows designed to release tension and ignite confidence. Even cooking nourishing meals for her family became a practice of honoring her body, her skills, and her choices.

Through each mindful sip, each stretch, and each quiet breath, Kyla remembered that her worth was not contingent on the mandates, the worries, or the expectations of others. Her worth was inherent. Unshakable.

By reclaiming her self-worth, Kyla didn't just stabilize herself; she modeled resilience and care for her children and her mother. She showed them that boundaries, mindfulness, and rituals of self-respect were not luxuries, they were lifelines.

Claiming Your Worth: The Kyla Way

Kyla's journey teaches us a vital truth: self-worth is not earned through sacrifice, compliance, or approval, it is remembered, reclaimed, and nurtured from within. Even in moments of fear, obligation, or overwhelm, small, intentional rituals of care anchor you in your own value.

As you enter the Self-Worth phase of your Confidence In Full Bloom journey, think of Kyla. Each morning tea, each mindful stretch, each pause to breathe is a seed. Water it consistently. Over time, those seeds grow into the quiet, unwavering belief that your worth is yours, simple, inherent, and unshakable.

Now it's your turn. Explore the Bloom At-Home Wellness practices and select one small ritual to start today. Which act of care will you add to your BYO Wellness Plan to honor your own inherent value?

Blooming Self – Worth: Daily Practice

"Confidence grows quietly in the soil of daily care."

Beautiful Bloomer, these first ten days are your grounding season, a return to calm, worth, and inner steadiness. You'll move through the **GROUND** cadence each day, simple acts that help your roots deepen.

Morning (G & R): Begin with **Gratitude** and **Reflection.** Start each day with your Bloom Essentials (See Appendix B:1a) - Sip your Revitalize Tea, stretch through Renew Yoga, and breathe in your Refresh Essential Oils Blend (or whatever is right to you). Feel your body awaken, your heart settle, your worth take hold.

Midday (O & U): Pause with **Openness** and **Uplift.** Step outside, notice something beautiful, or choose a **Bloom Booster** from your BYO worksheet. Let light and laughter refill your energy.

Evening (N & D): End with **Nurture** and **Declare or Dream.** Release the day with kindness. Whisper one truth of your worth before sleep: *I am enough. I am becoming.*

Keep your **Confidence in Full Bloom Journal**, pen, and Bloom Essentials close. These are your grow tools, your anchors, your reminders.

Each day that you cycle through GROUND, you'll remember what was never lost, just forgotten: your worth.

DAY 1: SEEDING VALUE

"A seed knows what it will become. It only needs light and time to grow."

Good morning, Radiant Bloomer. Today, we begin where all beauty begins, in the unseen. Beneath the surface, roots stir and whisper their quiet promises. So, it is with you. There is already something sacred growing in the soil of your being , your worth. It does not ask to be earned or proven, only remembered.

Take this day as an invitation to honor what already lives within you. The truth of your value is not a goal to chase; it is a garden waiting for your gentle tending.

MORNING RITUAL – Gratitude and Grounding

Begin your morning with your Bloom Essentials (Revitalize Tea, Renew Yoga, and Refresh Aromatherapy). Sip slowly. Let the warmth remind you that you are cared for.

Mantra: I am grateful for who I am.

Action: On a clean page in your *Confidence In Full Bloom Journal,* write down the qualities, gifts, and strengths that make you *you.* Don't rush. Let each word fall like a seed into soft earth.

Reflection: Ask yourself - How do these truths root you in self-worth?

MIDDAY RITUAL – Open and Uplift

Pause in the rhythm of your day. Step outside or stand by a window. Feel the air touch your skin , light, alive, and free.

Mantra: I open my heart to growth.

Action: Notice one small thing of beauty , a bird's flight, a shimmer of sunlight, a child's laughter. Let it lift you.

Reflection: In your journal, note how this moment of beauty shifted your energy.

EVENING RITUAL – Nurture and Declare

As twilight settles, return to stillness. Let the hum of the day fade, leaving only your breath and being.

Mantra: I rest in my worth.

Action: Read aloud your morning list of self-gratitudes. Let each word bloom again in the quiet.

Reflection: Ask yourself - How did declaring your truth feel in your body? Write freely.

CLOSING THOUGHT:

Today, you have planted a seed of remembrance that you were worthy before you ever began. Rest in that knowing and let tomorrow find you blooming.

DAY 2: PREPARING THE SOIL

"Before the bloom, there is the tending, the quiet work of care that roots us in possibility."

Good morning, Gorgeous Bloomer. Yesterday, you named your seeds , the truths and qualities that make you worthy. Today, we turn to the soil, the places within and around you where those seeds will take root. Every garden needs ground that breathes, soil that welcomes water and warmth. You, too, need an environment that honors your becoming.

Look closely at what surrounds you: the rooms you inhabit, the people who speak into your spirit, the thoughts that echo when the world grows still. Some things nourish. Others deplete. Preparing your soil means choosing to make space for what feeds you, safety, support, and light.

MORNING RITUAL – Grounding in Gratitude

Begin your day with your Bloom Essentials: Sip your Revitalize Tea, move through your Renew Yoga flow, breathe in your Refresh Aromatherapy blend. Feel the steadiness beneath your feet, the breath that connects you to this earth.

Mantra: I am grateful for the ground I stand on.

Action: On a clean page in your *Confidence In Full Bloom Journal,* list the spaces where you feel safe and supported. If none come easily, imagine them , a quiet corner, a café, a sunlit room, a garden bench. Let possibility itself be fertile ground.

Reflection: Ask yourself - How do safe spaces prepare me to grow?

MIDDAY RITUAL – Nourishing the Inner Garden

Pause for a moment of kindness toward yourself. Smile softly in the mirror; let it be real, not rushed. Choose one meal, snack, or sip that feels kind to your body , something that whispers “care” instead of “should.”

Mantra: I open my mind to new ways of caring for myself.

Action: Enjoy one nourishing food or drink with full attention. Taste the generosity in it.

Reflection: Ask yourself - How did this simple act shift my energy or mood? Write what you notice in your journal.

EVENING RITUAL – Rooted in Worthiness

As dusk settles, open your journal once more. Write a few “I am worthy” statements , truths that reclaim your dignity and quiet your doubt. Speak one aloud. Let your voice carry it into the room like incense.

Mantra: I dream of a life rooted in self-worth.

Action: Speak one “I am worthy” statement before sleep.

Reflection: Ask yourself - What worthiness truth will I carry into tomorrow?

CLOSING THOUGHT:

Tonight, you have tended the sacred ground of your becoming. The soil is richer now , layered with gratitude, gentleness, and truth. Rest in that goodness. Tomorrow will find you growing.

DAY 3: PLANTING INTENTION

"Intention is the quiet promise between your heart and your becoming."

Guten Tag (German), Graceful Bloomer. Yesterday, you prepared your soil , noticing the spaces where you feel safe, supported, and nourished. Today, you plant the seeds of intention, giving life to your strengths through mindful action. A gardener knows that planting is an act of faith , pressing hope into the earth before the bloom is visible. You, too, are planting what will one day rise and color your world.

Your kindness, creativity, patience, and curiosity are not abstract virtues; they are living seeds. When tended with awareness, they root themselves in your days , in your gestures, choices, and words. Each time you act with intention, you say to yourself, *"I am growing."*

MORNING RITUAL – Cultivating Strength

Begin your day with your Bloom Essentials , sip your Revitalize Tea, move through your Renew Yoga flow, breathe in your Refresh Aromatherapy blend. Let warmth, scent, and movement awaken your aliveness.

Mantra: I bring my strengths to life.

Action: On a clean page in your *Confidence In Full Bloom Journal,* choose one strength from your Day 1 list and plan a way to express it today.

– *Kindness:* Offer a genuine compliment or a patient ear.

–*Creativity:* Sketch, journal, or reimagine something familiar.

– *Patience:* Pause before reacting, breathe before speaking.

– *Curiosity:* Ask a question, explore, research, or simply wonder.

Reflection: Ask yourself - How will expressing this strength shape how I feel; in body, heart, and mind?

MIDDAY RITUAL – Nurturing Through Action

Find a quiet moment in your safe space. Notice the light, the sounds, the stillness, let them remind you that growth often begins in silence.

Mantra: I nurture my growth through action.

Action: Take one concrete step that reflects your chosen strength.

– *Kindness:* Offer a word of encouragement.

– *Creativity:* Try a new recipe or approach to a task.

– *Patience:* Listen fully without rushing the moment.

– *Curiosity:* Learn something new or explore an idea that sparks joy.

Reflection: How did this action shift my energy or sense of self-worth?

EVENING RITUAL – Honoring the Seeds

As night gathers, place a hand over your heart and take three deep breaths. Let gratitude settle where effort once stirred.

Mantra: I honor the seeds I have planted today.

Action: In your *Confidence In Full Bloom Journal,* note one way you expressed your strength in a safe or nurturing environment. Celebrate the smallest movement forward , it counts.

Reflection: Ask yourself - What did planting my intention teach me about my self-worth and my capacity to grow?

CLOSING THOUGHT:

Today, you placed your strengths gently into the soil of your life. Each mindful act is a promise , a whisper to your future self: *keep blooming.*

DAY 4: WATERING YOUR WORTH

"The garden does not grow from striving, but from steady love poured in small, faithful ways."

Buongiorno (Italian), Bright Bloomer. Yesterday, you planted the seeds of your strengths in safe and nourishing spaces. Today, you water those seeds. Watering your worth means giving attention, care, and energy to the truths you wish to grow. Just as a garden thrives through consistent tending, your self-worth deepens through moments of gratitude, presence, and gentle joy. Every act of care strengthens your roots and prepares you to bloom.

MORNING RITUAL – Gentle Gratitude

Begin your morning with your Bloom Essentials: sip your Revitalize Tea, move through your Renew Yoga flow, and breathe in your Refresh Aromatherapy blend. Feel warmth rise in your body and energy flow through your breath as you awaken to the day's quiet promise.

Mantra: I am watering the seeds of my worth.

Action: On a clean page in your *Confidence In Full Bloom Journal,* write three things you are grateful for today , moments, people, or qualities within yourself. As you write, imagine each gratitude as water falling onto your roots, nourishing your growth.

Reflection: Ask yourself - How does giving gratitude to myself support the growth of my self-worth?

MIDDAY RITUAL – Mindful Nourishment

Take five peaceful minutes to choose one *Emotional Wellness Bloom Booster* to nurture your worth. Options include Loving-Kindness Meditation, Nature Savoring or Forest Bathing, or a Music Ritual. Refer to your Bloom Booster list for details. Let this time be wholly yours.

Mantra: I nourish my worth with mindful care.

Action: Engage fully in your chosen Bloom Booster. Feel how this practice waters your inner garden, enriching the strengths you planted yesterday.

Reflection: Ask yourself - How does this practice make me feel in my body and heart? What does it reveal about my capacity to care for myself?

EVENING RITUAL – Rest and Renewal

Before bed, place a hand over your heart and take three slow, steady breaths. Visualize the personal qualities you've planted, being watered by your care , growing stronger with every act of kindness toward yourself.

Mantra: I rest knowing my worth is growing.

Action: Close your eyes and picture your inner garden flourishing. Speak one "I am worthy" statement from your list, slowly and with intention.

Reflection: Ask yourself - How does this visualization feel in my body? How does it strengthen my sense of self-worth?

CLOSING THOUGHT:

Today, you nourished your self-worth with gratitude and mindful attention. Each small act of care , a breath, a kindness, a moment of stillness , has watered the garden within. Trust that growth is already underway, quietly, and beautifully.

DAY 5: GERMINATING SELF -WORTH

"Growth is not loud or hurried. It happens quietly, where patience meets faith."

Sawubona (Zulu), Steady Bloomer. Yesterday, you nourished your worth with gratitude and mindful care. Today, you tend to the gentle unfolding of growth itself. Like tender shoots reaching for light, your intentions need room to stretch, breathe, and find their way. When you slow down, listen inward, and notice your progress without judgment, you give your self-worth space to take root in truth and clarity. Growth is not measured in leaps but in moments of awareness, kindness, and steady tending.

MORNING RITUAL – Awakening with Intention

Begin your day with your Bloom Essentials: sip your Revitalize Tea, move through your Renew Yoga flow, and breathe in your Refresh Aromatherapy blend. Let your morning light remind you that growth, like sunrise, is both gentle and inevitable.

Mantra: I create space for growth and clarity.

Action: Choose a Bloom Booster that feels nurturing today. As you engage, notice how the practice opens your mind or heart, giving your inner seed room to stretch and sprout.

Reflection: Ask yourself - How does this nurturing help my qualities grow stronger and more visible?

MIDDAY RITUAL – Tending with Awareness

Pause during your day to notice how you're growing in real time. Growth often hides in ordinary moments, how you speak to yourself, how you breathe through tension, how you choose peace over pressure. Give yourself a few quiet minutes to observe and honor what is unfolding.

Mantra: I honor my growth as it happens.

Action: Step away from your routine for a brief walk or still moment. As you move or breathe, name one small way you've grown this week.

Reflection: Ask yourself - How does acknowledging my progress help me stay rooted in trust and patience?

EVENING RITUAL – Nurture and Declare

Before bed, sit quietly and place your hand over your heart. Reflect on the growth you noticed today, no matter how small. Write a brief note of encouragement to yourself, as if speaking to a cherished friend, and read it aloud softly.

Mantra: I declare and honor my growth.

Action: Write one statement of encouragement and read it aloud slowly. For example: "I am courageous. I am creative. I am worthy."

Reflection: Ask yourself - How does this acknowledgment feel in my body? How does it reinforce the roots of my worth?

CLOSING THOUGHT:

Today, you have nurtured the quiet beginnings of growth. Your seed of self-worth is awakening, sending down roots, and reaching toward the light. Each mindful act, insight, and word of encouragement strengthens the foundation for your full bloom. You can be proud of how gently you're growing.

DAY 6: ROOTING SELF-WORTH

"Roots do their work in silence, holding us steady while we reach for the light."

Welcome back, Wise Bloomer. Yesterday, your seeds of self-worth began to stir beneath the surface, quietly waking to possibility. Today, you begin to root. Just as roots anchor a plant firmly into the earth, your values and truths ground you in strength and stability. Rooting means choosing what holds you steady, nourishes your being, and supports you through every season. When you live from your values, you create an unshakable foundation where your self-worth can thrive.

MORNING RITUAL – Grounded in Values

Begin your morning by centering yourself with your Bloom Essentials. Sip your warm tea, breathe in your grounding aromatherapy, and stretch through a slow, steady yoga flow that helps you feel the floor beneath you. Let each breath remind you of the earth's quiet support and your own inner steadiness.

Mantra: I am grateful for the roots that ground me.

Action: On a clean page in your *Confidence In Full Bloom Journal,* write down three values that feel like your personal roots , qualities such as honesty, compassion, faith, courage, or creativity.

Reflection: Ask yourself - How do these values support my sense of self-worth and give me strength?

MIDDAY RITUAL – Living Your Truth

At midday, strengthen your roots by putting one of your values into action. Choose an *Emotional Wellness Bloom Booster* from your list to support you in expressing it. Let your choices reflect what matters most to you.

Mantra: I rise tall because my roots are strong.

Action: Pick one value you named this morning and live it out in a small, deliberate way today.

Reflection: Ask yourself - How did practicing my value today make me feel more grounded and worthy?

EVENING RITUAL – Resting in Strength

As the day closes, settle into stillness. Sit quietly with your hand over your heart and breathe deeply. Feel how your body, mind, and spirit are held by the roots you've tended.

Mantra: I rest in the strength of my roots.

Action: Speak one of your values aloud three times, imagining it extending deeper into the soil of your being, drawing nourishment from truth.

Reflection: Ask yourself - Which value felt strongest in me today, and how did it nourish my sense of worth?

CLOSING THOUGHT:

Today, you rooted yourself more deeply in your foundation. Each value you claim and live becomes a root that steadies you through uncertainty and growth alike. Your self-worth draws strength from these roots, allowing you to rise with confidence and bloom with grace.

DAY 7: SPROUTING SELF-WORTH

"The moment you rise into the light, the world begins to see what was always waiting to bloom."

Konnichiwa (*Japanese*), Confident Bloomer. Today marks a tender turning point in your journey. Your seed of self-worth, long nurtured in stillness, begins to emerge. Sprouting is the quiet miracle of becoming visible when what was hidden beneath the surface dares to meet the light. It is courage made flesh, truth given form. You may feel delicate, but there is immense power in this stage. The sprout does not question its right to rise; it simply reaches. This is your day to practice showing yourself to the world with gentleness, courage, and grace.

MORNING RITUAL – Courage to Emerge

Begin your day with your Bloom Essentials: sip your warm tea, breathe in your grounding aromatherapy, and stretch through a slow yoga flow that wakes your body with care. Let gratitude be the sunlight that greets your first thought.

Mantra: I am grateful for my courage to emerge.

Action: On a clean page in your *Confidence In Full Bloom Journal,* write one area of your life where you are beginning to show more of yourself, at work, at home, or simply in how you move through your day.

Reflection: Ask yourself - How does it feel to let myself be seen here?

MIDDAY RITUAL – Opening to Light

Growth requires space, and so do you. Take a few moments to step into the light, literally or figuratively. Choose a *Bloom Booster* that refreshes your spirit, whether it's fresh air, gentle movement, or a quiet pause with tea. Then, meet your own eyes in the mirror. Let presence be your affirmation.

Mantra: I open myself to visibility.

Action: Smile softly at your reflection, allowing that moment of connection to affirm your worth.

Reflection: Ask yourself - How did this small act uplift my confidence?

EVENING RITUAL – Resting in Visibility

As night falls, settle into stillness. Like a sprout resting after stretching toward the sun, you, too, can rest in the truth that you are growing. Speak to yourself kindly, acknowledging the courage it takes to be seen.

Mantra: I declare my right to be seen.

Action: Whisper gently to yourself, "My worth is visible."

Reflection: Ask yourself - Where did I shine today?

CLOSING THOUGHT:

Today, you honored your emergence. By tending your Bloom Essentials, nurturing your energy, and daring to be visible, you stepped into the light with quiet confidence. Your sprout grows stronger with every act of authenticity. Keep rising, you were made for this light.

DAY 8: GROWING WITH JOY

"Growth is not a race; it is a rhythm, a quiet unfolding of grace meeting intention."

Bonjour *(In a French accent),* Joyful Bloomer. Today, your sprout begins to grow. Growth is a dance between effort and ease, awareness, and rest. It isn't hurried or measured by comparison, it happens moment by moment, breath by breath. Growing with joy means showing up for yourself in love, not pressure. It means choosing kindness over criticism, intention over autopilot, and gratitude over doubt. You are learning to flourish from within, reminding yourself daily that you are worthy of this becoming.

MORNING RITUAL – Grateful Awareness

Begin your morning with your Bloom Essentials. Brew a warm cup of tea, move through gentle yoga stretches, and awaken your senses with aromatherapy. Let your breath be your guide back to presence and feel the quiet steadiness of being alive.

Mantra: I am grateful for my progress.

Action: On a clean page in your *Confidence In Full Bloom Journal,* list three things you accomplished this past week, no matter how small. Each one is proof of your persistence and your care.

Reflection: Ask yourself - How do these accomplishments reflect my worth?

MIDDAY RITUAL – Open to Lightness

At midday, feed your growth with energy and joy. Step outside for a few minutes of fresh air, enjoy a colorful piece of fruit, or move your body with intention. Choose a *Bloom Booster* that brings play or delight into your day. Movement and laughter are water for the soul.

Mantra: I open to growth opportunities.

Action: Take a mindful walk or stretch for five minutes, breathing in rhythm with your movement.

Reflection: Ask yourself - How does this moment of movement or openness support my growth?

EVENING RITUAL – Resting in Worth

As your day comes to a close, return to stillness. Growth also happens in rest, in the pause between one breath and the next. Speak a gentle affirmation of worth aloud, allowing your body to soften into its truth.

Mantra: I rest in my worth.

Action: Speak one affirmation aloud, such as "I am growing beautifully," and let it settle into your spirit as you relax into rest.

Reflection: Ask yourself - How does this affirmation feel physically and emotionally?

CLOSING THOUGHT:

Today, you nourished your growth with gratitude, movement, and presence. Each step forward, each breath of awareness, each moment of joy carries you closer to your full bloom. Growth doesn't demand proof; it only asks that you keep showing up in love.

DAY 9: STEMMING SELF-WORTH UPWARDS

"Strength is not in rushing to bloom, but in learning how to rise with grace."

Goeie dag (Afrikaans), Grand Bloomer. Today, your growth moves upward. Just as a flower's stem carries water and light to nourish the bloom, your stem represents the inner structure that lifts your self-worth into visibility. Stemming upward is the practice of alignment, of letting your confidence, care, and purpose rise through steady, intentional living. Each choice to nurture your energy, honor your rhythm, and move with joy strengthens your inner stem. Over time, you'll notice that what once felt heavy becomes lighter, and what once seemed far away begins to come within reach.

MORNING RITUAL – Rising with Intention

Begin your morning by pouring into yourself so that you can rise with strength. Brew your tea and breathe in the steam as it curls upward, a symbol of your own ascent. Move through gentle yoga stretches that lengthen your body and diffuse an aroma that helps you feel both grounded and uplifted. Let each movement remind you that energy, like self-worth, flows best when given care and space.

Mantra: I am grateful for the beauty preparing to bloom.

Action: On a clean page in your *Confidence In Full Bloom Journal,* write one thing you're anticipating with joy.

Reflection: Ask yourself - How does looking forward feel in my body?

MIDDAY RITUAL – Opening to Possibility

As the day unfolds, remind yourself that your inner stem carries you upward with every breath and choice. Take a brief pause and visualize one possibility that excites you, something you hope to experience or create. See it clearly, as though it already exists, and allow your spirit to respond.

Mantra: I open to what's coming.

Action: Close your eyes for three minutes and visualize your possibility in vivid detail. Then, write what you saw in your journal.

Reflection: Ask yourself - How does imagining my possibilities make me feel?

EVENING RITUAL – Rooted and Ready

As the evening settles, bring your awareness to the strength that has been building within you. Place a hand over your heart and feel your own steady pulse, proof that life is still moving upward, still believing in your bloom.

Mantra: I declare my readiness.

Action: Before sleep, softly say, "I am ready to bloom."

Reflection: Ask yourself - What stirred in me today?

CLOSING THOUGHT:

Each action you took today helped your self-worth rise a little higher. You are building your strength, balance, and flow, steadying yourself for the bloom that is already forming. You are growing taller, stronger, and more ready with every breath of intention.

DAY 10: BLOOMING SELF- WORTH

"To bloom is to remember that you were beautiful all along, simply waiting for the right light to unfold."

Bula Vinaka (Fijian), Beautiful Bloomer. Today, if you are ready, you are invited to open fully into the light of who you are. Blooming is not about perfection or performance; it is the natural expression of care, patience, and devotion. You have tended your soil, watered your roots, and reached toward the sun. Now, your worth stands revealed, radiant, alive, and deserving of celebration. Blooming is your declaration that you are enough, exactly as you are, and that your becoming is worthy of joy.

MORNING RITUAL – Grateful Unfolding

Begin your day with your Bloom Essentials. Sip your tea slowly, move through gentle yoga stretches, and breathe in your favorite aromatherapy scent. Let each ritual remind you of how far you've come and how naturally you continue to grow.

Mantra: I am grateful for the fullness of who I am.

Action: On a clean page in your *Confidence In Full Bloom Journal,* write three ways you are already blooming in your life. Notice how good it feels to name them.

Reflection: Ask yourself - How can I celebrate myself today? List a few ways in your journal.

MIDDAY RITUAL – Opening to Joy

Growth continues through joy and lightness. Take time today to celebrate your progress, however it appears. Step outside, turn your face toward the sun, dance for a moment, or enjoy a sweet treat that feels like delight itself.

Mantra: I open to joy and fulfillment.

Action: Choose one small act of celebration from your list and do it with intention. If possible, take a brief walk and notice something in nature that is also blooming, a flower, a tree, or even the sky.

Reflection: Ask yourself - How did my act of celebration uplift my spirit?

EVENING RITUAL – Resting in Radiance

As the day quiets, turn inward and honor your bloom. Place a hand over your heart and breathe deeply, allowing the truth of your worth to settle in your body.

Mantra: I dream forward in my worth.

Action: Speak softly to yourself: "I am blooming in my worth."

Reflection: Ask yourself - What truth about my worth will carry me onward?

CLOSING THOUGHT:

Today, you celebrated your bloom. To bloom is to honor your growth in every season, to know that your worth has never needed proof, only your attention. Each act of recognition and joy strengthens your light. Stand tall in this beauty, Beautiful Bloomer. You are the garden come alive.

Self-Worth: Closing Summary

"To know your worth is to return home to yourself, to the quiet knowing that you are already enough."

Congratulations, Confident Bloomer. You've completed the foundational ten-day journey of Self-Worth, planting the first seeds of confidence, self-recognition, and emotional resilience. Over these days, you tended the soil of your being with patience and intention. You've moved from rooting yourself in gratitude and awareness to sprouting visibility, strength, and readiness to bloom.

This phase followed the **GROUND Bloomprint cadence**, guiding you through daily rhythms that helped you remember your value in mind, body, and spirit:

Morning – Gratitude and Reflection: Each sunrise invited you to notice the good, journal your accomplishments, and reflect on what strengthens your self-worth.

Midday – Open and Uplift: These pauses lifted your spirit through movement, joy, and small intentional acts that nourished your emotional and mental well-being.

Evening – Nurture and Declare: Each night you affirmed your worth, visualized your growth, and acknowledged your efforts, allowing truth to take root where doubt once lived.

Your **Bloom At-Home Emotional and Mental Wellness practices** anchored this phase: journaling, reflection, mindfulness, visualization, affirmations, and celebrating your small wins. Through these simple but sacred rituals, you strengthened your self-awareness, emotional resilience, and your capacity to honor your intrinsic worth.

Through this journey, you learned to:

- Acknowledge and celebrate your daily victories, no matter how small.
- Cultivate gratitude and mindfulness as anchors for your sense of self.
- Nurture your confidence and visibility as you move toward deeper self-expression and empowerment.

This phase taught you that **self-worth isn't given; it's cultivated.** It grows through awareness, reflection, and intentional recognition of your progress. By grounding yourself in gratitude, openness, and affirmation, you've built a strong foundation for everything to come.

Carry forward the spirit of **GROUND**: give thanks freely, reflect deeply, open your heart to joy, nurture your mind and emotions, and declare your value daily. Each act of care reinforces your worth and prepares you to thrive in every dimension of life.

You should be deeply proud of yourself, Beautiful Bloomer. You have laid the foundation for all that comes next.

When you're ready, complete your **Post-Blooming Self-Worth Quick Assessment** to see where you stand after ten days of tending your emotional wellness and remembering your worth.

And when you turn the page, Phase 2 awaits, where Self-Efficacy begins to grow from everything you've planted here.

Post - Blooming Self-Worth Quick Assessment

Instructions: For each statement, rate yourself from **1 (Not at all true)** to **5 (Completely true).** Tally your score at the end and compare to Day 1.

Part 1: Quick Self-Check

		1-5
1	I take daily actions that uplift my mood or energy.	
2	I celebrate small wins in my life.	
3	I practice gratitude regularly.	
4	I feel supported and connected to others.	
5	I notice and embrace joy in my daily life.	
6	I speak my truth with honesty and compassion.	
7	I feel proud of who I am becoming.	
8	I believe in my own value and worth.	
9	I feel confident expressing my true self.	
	Total	

Part 2: Blooming Reflections:

What shifted most for me over the last 10 days?

Which practice(s) felt the most empowering for me?

Part 3: My Victory Statement

In your journal, write a short declaration that celebrates your blooming.

Post Emotional Wellness Check-in: Shade and name the pie.

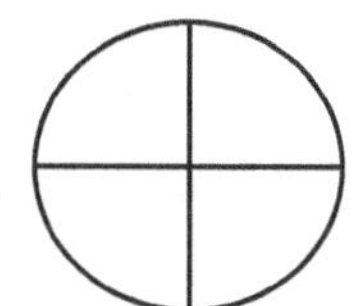

My current state:

Blooming Reflection: The Bridge Between Being and Believing

> Once, there was a woman who carried a cracked clay jar to gather water at the river each morning.
>
> Every day she filled it to the brim, and every day, by the time she reached home, most of the water had leaked away.
>
> She grew ashamed of her jar. She thought, If I were stronger, if I were better, I could hold it all together.
>
> Then one morning, as the sun rose, she noticed wildflowers blooming along her path, tiny bursts of color where her jar had dripped.
>
> The crack that once embarrassed her had been watering life, creating beauty all along.
>
> That day, she stopped wishing to be whole and started recognizing her worth, just as she was.
>
> She filled her jar again, no longer afraid of what might spill, but knowing she was meant to pour it freely.
>
> That's the bridge between self-worth and self-efficacy: the moment you stop hiding what's imperfect and start using it with purpose.

Phase 2:

Blooming Self-Efficacy

You are off to a beautiful blooming start. This new phase is where your roots deepen, and your victory stems begin to grow upward. Growth isn't just about movement, it's about direction, intention, and resilience.

Anchor List for Phase 2

1. Take Your Self-Efficacy & Physical Wellness Assessments - Awareness is the first act of confidence.
2. Create Your BYO Bloom-At-Home Wellness Plan- Choose rituals and rhythms that help you feel grounded and nourished each day.
3. Meet Allegra - Your Phase 2 story
4. companion.
5. Practice Self-Efficacy – Set goals
6. and achieve them.

Blooming Self-Efficacy Quick Assessments

SELF-EFFICACY ASSESSMENT

Instructions: For each statement, rate yourself from **1 (Not at all true)** to **5 (Completely true).** Total your points at the end.

Part 1: Inner Beliefs

		1-5
1	I feel confident in my ability to reach my goals.	
2	I trust myself to take consistent action.	
3	I can handle challenges and adapt when needed.	

Part 2: Daily Habits

		1-5
4	I set and track physical or wellness goals regularly.	
5	I take deliberate action to move my body and care for my wellness.	
6	I use available resources (tools, apps, support) to help me succeed.	

Part 3: Growth & Resilience in Action

		1-5
7	I celebrate small victories along the way.	
8	I stay motivated to continue my wellness practices even when busy.	
9	I feel a sense of accomplishment from completing wellness actions.	

Total	

Blooming Self-Efficacy Quick Assessment – Key

- **9–18:** Your self-efficacy garden is just sprouting. This 10-day journey will help you build strong new stems of confidence in action.
- **19–31:** You already have green shoots of self-efficacy. Over the next 10 days, you'll strengthen and stretch them toward the sun.
- **32–45**: You carry a thriving sense of self-efficacy. Use this journey to deepen your resilience and expand your flourishing.

PHYSICAL WELLNESS CHECK AND GOAL SETTING

This reflective exercise helps you assess your current physical wellness and set realistic goals for growth during your Self-Efficacy phase. You'll return to this same page on Day 10 to notice your progress and celebrate your wins.

What This Measures

Your physical wellness pie represents how effectively you're supporting your body as you build confidence and trust in your ability to follow through. Consider:

- How consistently you're caring for your physical needs (sleep, hydration, nourishment, movement)
- How your energy levels align with your daily actions and goals

- How much physical tension or fatigue comes from emotional stress or self-doubt
- How movement or body awareness helps you feel capable and strong

Instructions

Step 1: Measure Your Current Wellness: Look at the pie chart divided into four quarters (each worth 25% for a total of 100%). Using a colored pencil, crayon, or marker, shade in the amount that represents your physical wellness TODAY.

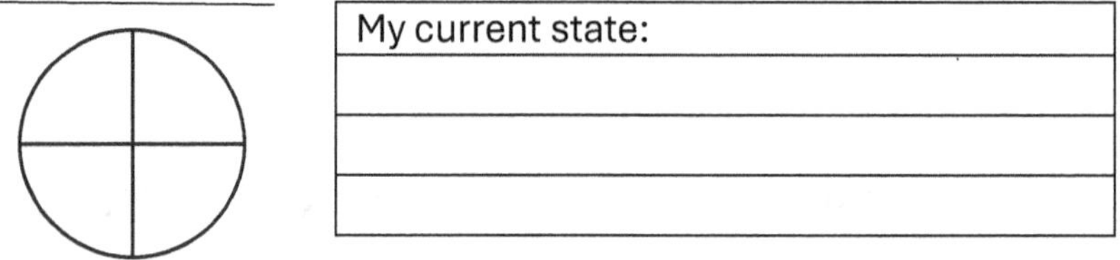

Shading Guide:

- 4 full quarters (100%) – You feel energized, well-rested, and physically aligned with your goals.
- 3 full quarters (75%) – You feel mostly well, with only minor stress or fatigue showing up.
- 2 full quarters (50%) – You notice some physical strain or inconsistency but are managing.
- 1 full quarter (25%) – Stress, fatigue, or lack of movement are significantly impacting your energy.
- No shading (0%) – Your body feels depleted or disconnected from your confidence-building efforts.

- Partial quarters: Shade portions of a quarter to represent a more precise percentage.

Example: If you feel your physical wellness is at about 37%, you would completely shade 1 quarter (25%) and shade half of a second quarter (12%).

Step 2: Name Your Current State: On the line above your shaded pie, write a name that captures how you feel physically right now.

Examples of naming:

- Learning to Listen to My Body"
- "Tired but Taking Action"
- "Finding My Strength Again"
- "Calm, Grounded, and Capable"

Step 3: Explain Current State: Next to your pie, write 2-3 sentences describing:

- **Points of strength:** What's working well physically? Where do you feel progress or vitality?
- **Points of challenge**: What needs more attention? How is stress or self-doubt showing up in your body?

Example: "I've been more consistent with stretching and hydration (strength), but I still wake up tense in my shoulders and tend to skip meals when I'm anxious about getting everything done (challenge)."

Step 4: Set Your 10-Day Goal

In the space provided, shade a second pie showing where you hope your physical wellness will be after ten days of focused self-efficacy practice. This becomes your target for the next ten days, your proof of progress.

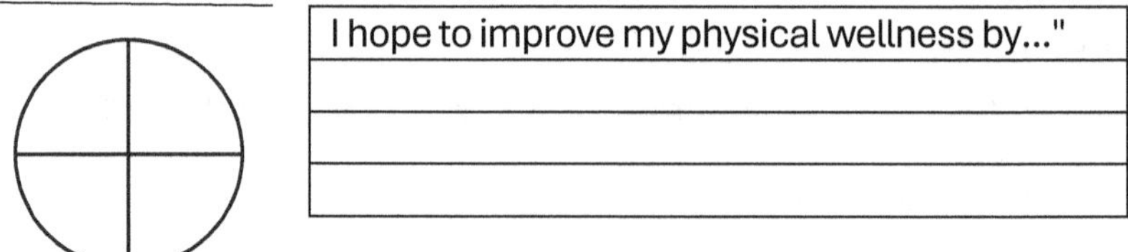

Step 5: Write Your Intention

Complete this sentence: "Over the next 10 days, I hope to improve my physical wellness by..."

Examples:

- "...creating a simple morning movement routine to boost my energy and confidence."
- "...maintaining consistent sleep and meal patterns, even on stressful days."
- "...practicing deep breathing or stretching when I feel tense instead of pushing through."
- "...tracking my energy levels and celebrating the small ways my body supports me."

BYO Bloom At-Home Physical Wellness Plan

This is your moment to design a wellness plan that speaks to your soul. See Appendices B:2a and B:2b. Choose the Bloom At-Home Wellness practices that call to you. What helps you feel grounded, peaceful, safe, and whole? There's no right or wrong. Let your heart and health lead you. Use the space below to build you plan:

Plan 1

Sunrise	
Midday	
Bedtime	

Plan 2

Sunrise	
Midday	
Bedtime	

Plan 3

Sunrise	
Midday	
Bedtime	

ALLEGRA'S STORY: The Power of Setting Goals

Allegra sat at her desk long after everyone else had gone home, the glow of her computer screen casting sharp light across stacks of files. The layoffs had hit her law firm hard, and the "lucky ones" left behind were drowning in double workloads.

She used to find comfort in routine, but now even that betrayed her, early mornings, skipped lunches, late nights answering emails marked *urgent.*

She'd started to call it *"the quiet burnout."*

No one talked about it, but everyone felt it.

Her husband urged her to stay put.

"Just ride it out," he'd say. "It's a good job." " We can't risk anything right now, not with the economy the way it is."

He wasn't wrong. But every day, Allegra felt herself fading , like watercolor left too long in the sun. Her creative energy was gone, her shoulders ached from stress, and she woke up every morning with a dull knot behind her ribs that whispered, *This can't be all there is.*

One morning, while refilling her coffee for the third time before 9 a.m., she caught her reflection in the microwave door: pale, tired, hunched. Something inside her snapped , softly, but decisively.

She couldn't control the economy. She couldn't fix the layoffs. But she could take one small step toward feeling alive again.

That night, she set a single goal: move her body every day for 10 minutes.

No gym membership. No pressure. Just movement.

She started with a simple goal to stretch each day. She began stretching on the living room floor after dinner, soft music playing, her breath syncing with her body again. Within a week, she was walking around the block. A month later, she was waking up early to do yoga before work, the morning sun spilling across her mat like a quiet promise that she still belonged to herself.

Those initial 10 minutes became a doorway. Her body began to feel stronger. Her mind, clearer. She stopped reacting to every crisis email like it was a fire and started pacing her day; breathe, stretch, and respond.

She noticed something: when she honored small goals the strengthened her body, she could manage bigger ones at work.

Her focus sharpened. Her tone steadied.

She stopped apologizing in meetings for things that weren't her fault.

And outside of work?

She pulled out her sketchbook again, setting a SMART creativity goal to draw one new piece a week. The same discipline that helped her stretch her body began to stretch her confidence. Each small win became proof that she wasn't stuck; she was rebuilding herself from the inside out.

When her husband noticed the changes , her energy, her mood, the way she carried herself , he finally said, "You seem different. Happier."

Allegra shared. "I just started keeping the promises I make to myself."

The job didn't change overnight. The world didn't either. But Allegra did.

And that was enough to shift everything.

Building Self-Efficacy, the Allegra Way

Allegra's story reminds us that self-efficacy , the belief that you can plan, act, and succeed , doesn't begin with a grand plan or a perfect opportunity. It begins with one decision: to show up for yourself.

In a VUCA world, control is rare. But you can always control your *effort.*

When Allegra started setting small physical goals , ten minutes of movement, a few mindful breaths, one page in her sketchbook , she wasn't just improving her health. She was proving to herself that she could follow through, even under pressure.

That's the essence of self-efficacy:

Consistency over chaos. Progress over perfection. It's how we learn to trust ourselves again , one action at a time.

So today, don't wait for stability to appear. Create it through small, intentional goals that strengthen your body and your belief in yourself.

Because once you realize you can move your body, you'll remember that you can move your life too.

Blooming Self – Efficacy: Daily Practice

“Confidence builds quietly each time you move with intention.”

Beautiful Bloomer, these next ten days are your growing season , a time to strengthen trust in yourself through small, steady action. You’ll move through the **GROW** cadence each day: Goals, Resourcefulness, Ownership, and Wins , practices that turn motion into confidence.

Morning (G): Begin with your **Bloom Essentials** , sip your Recharge Herbal Tea, stretch through your Rise Yoga Sequence, and breathe in your Resilient Essential Oils Blend from Appendix B:2a. As your body awakens, set one clear, achievable goal for the day. Let intention be your morning fuel.

Midday (R & O): Pause with purpose. Notice your energy and use your **Bloom Boosters** from Appendix B:2b to refocus , take a mindful walk, hydrate, stretch, or ask for help when needed. Honor your progress and take ownership of how you move forward.

Evening (W): Wind down with reflection. Note what you accomplished, however small, and whisper: *I’m proud of what I built today.*

Keep your **Confidence in Full Bloom Journal**, pen, and Bloom Essentials close.

Each day through **GROW**, you strengthen your muscles, body, mind, and belief in yourself, one intentional movement at a time.

DAY 1 – PLANTING SELF-EFFICACY: SIMPLE GOALS

"Confidence grows not from grand gestures, but from the quiet courage to begin again each day."

Good day to you, Glorious Bloomer. Today, you plant the first seed of self-efficacy by setting a simple goal. A simple goal is a promise you make to yourself, clear, manageable, and meaningful enough to move you forward. Growth begins here, in small, deliberate steps. Each time you choose to act, to follow through, and to celebrate the doing, you build trust in your own ability to shape your life. These little acts of faith in yourself are how confidence takes root and begins to rise.

MORNING RITUAL – Goals and Resourcefulness

Begin your day with your Bloom Essentials , sip your Recharge Tea, move gently through your Rise Yoga flow, and breathe in your Resilient Aromatherapy blend. As your body awakens, turn your attention to one simple goal you can complete today. Let it be something attainable yet meaningful: a five-minute stretch, a short walk, or drinking an extra glass of water. Picture yourself completing it and notice how your body responds to that vision of success.

Mantra: I can achieve simple goals.

Action: On a clean page in your *Confidence In Full Bloom Journal,* write one small “physical wellness” goal for today , something doable, personal, and purposeful.

Reflection: Ask yourself - What resources, time, or support do I have to succeed in this goal today?

MIDDAY RITUAL – Ownership and Momentum

At midday, pause to check in with yourself. Even small actions matter. They remind you that you are capable of directing your day and influencing your experience. By noticing your progress, you affirm your ability to create change.

Mantra: I own my choice to move forward.

Action: Complete your simple goal, whether during a break, at home, or in motion between tasks. Let it feel like a gift to yourself.

Reflection: Ask yourself - How did taking responsibility to complete my goal feel in my body?

EVENING RITUAL – Recognizing Wins

As night gathers, take a few moments to honor what you've done today. Every small win is a declaration of self-belief, a whisper that says, *I can.* Reflect on your effort, not its size, and feel how accomplishment softens and strengthens you at once.

Mantra: I celebrate every step.

Action: In your *Confidence In Full Bloom Journal,* write down one small win from today , no matter how minor it may seem.

Reflection: Ask yourself - How does recognizing this achievement motivate me to take the next step?

CLOSING THOUGHT: Today, you planted the first seed of self-efficacy and tended it with intention. Through one clear action, you began the process of trusting yourself to do what you say you will do. This is how confidence grows, through the simple rhythm of trying, doing, and celebrating. Keep showing up for yourself, Glorious Bloomer. You are building strength one choice at a time.

DAY 2 – WATERING SELF-EFFICACY: CONSISTENCY AND CARE

"Growth doesn't rush, it trusts. Every drop of effort counts when you keep showing up for yourself."

Aloha (Polynesian), Almighty Bloomer. Yesterday, you planted your first seed of self-efficacy by setting a simple goal. Today, you water that seed with consistency. Just as a plant depends on steady rain to grow strong, your confidence thrives on repetition and care. Each time you return to your goal, showing up, following through, and tending your progress, you teach yourself reliability. You prove that you can be trusted with your own becoming.

MORNING RITUAL – Rooted in Routine

Begin your day with your Bloom Essentials, your Recharge Tea, move gently through your Rise Yoga flow, and breathe in your Resilient Aromatherapy blend. Let the rhythm of your morning remind you that consistency doesn't have to be complicated; it's simply devotion in motion.

Mantra: Consistency grows my strength.

Action: In your *Confidence In Full Bloom Journal,* repeat and expand yesterday's goal. Add one extra minute, one new repetition, or one small refinement. Let this new layer of effort become your next step.

Reflection: Ask yourself - Which tools or supports will help me stay consistent today?

MIDDAY RITUAL – Owning the Process

Pause in the heart of your day to give yourself a little "sunlight." Choose a *Bloom Booster* that reenergizes your body and spirit, step outside for fresh air, take a mindful walk, savor a bright piece of fruit, or try box breathing. Each choice is a way of saying; *I am responsible for my growth.*

Mantra: I take responsibility for my progress.

Action: Track your goal's progress visibly, in your journal, planner, or app. Let yourself see your effort take shape.

Reflection: Ask yourself - How does taking ownership of my progress increase my confidence?

EVENING RITUAL – Honoring the Effort

As the evening settles, turn inward and honor the quiet power of your follow-through. Even when growth feels subtle, it is happening. Celebrate your effort as evidence of your commitment.

Mantra: I honor my commitment.

Action: Record your completed goal as a win in your *Confidence In Full Bloom Journal.*

Reflection: Ask yourself - How does acknowledging effort feel in my body?

CLOSING THOUGHT:

Today, you watered your seed with consistency and care. Each small act strengthened your trust in yourself and deepened your roots of self-efficacy. Keep returning to your goals with patience and presence, the garden of your confidence is growing, one intentional day at a time.

DAY 3 – ROOTING SELF-EFFICACY: STRETCHING INTO GROWTH

"Confidence deepens when you dare to reach beyond the familiar, steady enough to wobble, brave enough to grow."

Glad tidings (Old English) Gregarious Bloomer. Over the past two days, you've planted and watered your simple goals. Today, you root deeper by stretching , adding just a little variety, a touch more reach, a gentle challenge to what you've already begun. Just as roots push through the soil seeking strength and nourishment, you too expand by exploring what lies just beyond comfort. Growth loves curiosity; it responds beautifully when you meet it halfway.

MORNING RITUAL – Expanding with Intention

Begin your day with your Bloom Essentials , sip your Recharge Tea, flow through your Rise Yoga sequence, and breathe in your Resilient Aromatherapy blend. Let your body and breath remind you that expansion doesn't mean overwhelm; it means willingness.

Mantra: I am open to growing stronger through small stretches.

Action: Add a small variation to your simple goal's routine. Walk the stairs instead of the hall, dance for five minutes, or try a brief desk yoga session. Choose one way to gently ramp up your effort.

Reflection: Ask yourself – What new resources or supports will help me sustain this stretch in my growth?

MIDDAY RITUAL – Ownership in Motion

As you move through your day, notice how it feels to go beyond your usual rhythm. Trying something new strengthens both your body and your confidence. Rooting takes ownership , your steady, intentional hand watering your own progress. Each time you say yes to your growth, you declare your readiness to rise.

Mantra: I own my choice to stretch further.

Action: Complete your expanded goal and mark it as done in your *Confidence In Full Bloom Journal.* Celebrate the follow-through.

Reflection: Ask yourself – In what way did exploring and expanding my goal make me feel more empowered?

EVENING RITUAL – Honoring Adaptability

Tonight, reflect on how you stretched today. Recognizing your adaptability reinforces your self-trust , the quiet knowing that you can handle change and growth with grace. Every acknowledgment deepens your roots of confidence.

Mantra: I celebrate adaptability.

Action: In your journal, note your first "stretching" win of Phase 2.

Reflection: Ask yourself – How does this small act of adaptability reinforce my belief in my own capability?

CLOSING THOUGHT:

Today, you rooted your confidence in new experiences, strengthening your foundation for continued growth. What began as a simple goal has now become proof of your consistency, courage, and adaptability. Each small stretch is a step toward mastery , a deeper trust in what you can do and who you're becoming.

Tomorrow, you'll begin shaping your goals with structure and clarity through SMART goals , giving your growing confidence a framework to flourish. Rest easy, Beautiful Bloomer. You've earned this calm before the next bloom.

DAY 4 – PLANTING SELF-EFFICACY: SMART GOALS

"Clarity is kindness to your future self. Each defined step is a promise you keep with your own becoming."

Grand rising, (Caribbean) Carful Bloomer. Today, you plant a SMART goal , a clear and structured seed that will guide your growth. While simple goals helped you practice consistency, SMART goals give your confidence a framework, turning good intentions into tangible direction. SMART stands for *Specific, Measurable, Achievable, Relevant,* and *Time-bound.* Each part helps you set goals that are realistic, motivating, and trackable , goals that make your progress visible, one step at a time.

Instead of saying, *"I'll exercise more,"* a SMART goal might sound like: *"I will walk for 10 minutes after lunch for the next three days."* This kind of clarity gives your growth something to hold onto , structure, rhythm, and purpose. Today, you're not just setting a goal; you're learning to trust the process that will carry you forward.

MORNING RITUAL – Goals and Resourcefulness

Begin your day with your Bloom Essentials , sip your Recharge Herbal Tea, stretch through your Rise Yoga Sequence, and breathe in your Resilient Essential Oils Blend. These morning rituals awaken your energy and clear your mind for focused intention. When you feel grounded, bring your attention to a goal that supports your physical wellness , one that feels achievable within the next few days.

Mantra: Clarity strengthens my growth.

Action: In your *Confidence In Full Bloom Journal,* write one SMART physical wellness goal you can accomplish soon. For example: *"I* *will complete 10 squats after breakfast each morning for the next three days."*

Reflection: Ask yourself – What supports or strategies can help me take this goal step by step?

Sample Physical Wellness SMART Goals:

1. *Walking Goal* – "I will walk for 20 minutes, three times per week, for the next month."
2. *Hydration Goal* – "I will drink at least 8 cups (64 ounces) of water each day for the next two weeks."
3. *Strength Goal* – "I will complete 2 strength-training sessions per week, lasting at least 30 minutes, for the next six weeks."
4. *Sleep Goal* – "I will go to bed by 10:30 p.m. on weeknights for the next three weeks."
5. *Stretching Goal* – "I will stretch for 5 minutes each morning after waking for the next 14 days."
6. *Screen-Time Reset* – "I will unplug from devices 30 minutes before bed, 5 nights a week, for the next month."

MIDDAY RITUAL – Ownership and Momentum

At midday, pause to check in with your energy. Notice your willingness to follow through. Ownership is power , the quiet kind that grows with every deliberate choice. To stay energized, use a *Physical Wellness Bloom Booster* such as a brisk walk, desk yoga, or deep breathing.

Mantra: I own my commitment to measurable growth.

Action: Begin your SMART goal today with one small step and record your progress in your *Confidence In Full Bloom Journal.*

Reflection: Ask yourself – How does ownership feel when I approach my goal step by step?

EVENING RITUAL – Honoring Clear Progress

As the day softens, look back on your progress with pride. Wins don't need to be big to be meaningful. Every measurable action , even writing the goal itself , reinforces your ability to plan, act, and achieve.

Mantra: I celebrate clear progress.

Action: Record your measurable achievement in your *Confidence In Full Bloom Journal.* Write down what you completed , minutes walked, stretches held, or actions begun.

Reflection: Ask yourself – How does acknowledging these small steps build my confidence and motivation?

CLOSING THOUGHT:

Today, you planted a SMART goal with clarity and care. By defining your steps and honoring your follow-through, you've given your growth direction and depth. Each clear action strengthens your self-efficacy, reminding you that you are capable, disciplined, and beautifully becoming.

Tomorrow, you'll expand this SMART goal , breaking it into smaller, steady actions that help your confidence take deeper root. Rest well, Superstar. You're learning to lead your own growth with grace.

DAY 5 – WATERING SELF-EFFICACY: SMART GOALS IN ACTION

"Big change begins with small, faithful steps. Every simple action is a whisper that says, I believe in my becoming."

Salutations, Sassy Bloomer. Yesterday, you planted a SMART goal , something clear, meaningful, and achievable. Today, you water that goal by breaking it down into smaller, doable steps. Growth happens when dreams meet structure, when clarity is followed by gentle, consistent action. Dividing your goal into simple steps makes it less daunting and turns each day into a chance to celebrate progress.

MORNING RITUAL – Goals and Resourcefulness

Begin your day with your Bloom Essentials , sip your Recharge Herbal Tea, stretch through your Rise Yoga Sequence, and breathe in your Resilient Essential Oils Blend. Let your body wake with purpose. Then, bring your focus to your SMART goal. Break it into one or two smaller tasks that feel realistic and kind to your current energy.

Mantra: I adjust and break tasks into steps.

Action: Identify a few small, actionable steps that lead you toward your SMART goal. Write them in your *Confidence In Full Bloom Journal.*

Reflection: Ask yourself – Which resources can I use to make completing these steps easier?

Examples of SMART Goal Steps:

• *If your SMART goal is to walk three mornings a week for 20 minutes*, your first step could be setting out your shoes and workout clothes each night.

• *If your SMART goal is to cook healthy dinners three times this week*, start by selecting recipes or making your grocery list.

• *If your SMART goal is to journal before bed four nights this week*, your step might be placing your journal and pen on your nightstand and setting a reminder on your phone.

Each small step waters your goal and helps it grow stronger. Layer in your Bloom Boosters , a favorite song, gratitude, or a joyful pause , to keep the process light and alive.

MIDDAY RITUAL – Ownership and Focus

Pause midday and notice how it feels to act on your smaller tasks. Each one you complete is a vote of confidence in your ability to follow through. Taking ownership of your progress reinforces your self-efficacy and your trust in your own rhythm.

Mantra: I take responsibility for each step I take.

Action: Complete one or more of your smaller steps today, focusing on one at a time. When you finish, use a Bloom Booster , perhaps a stretch, a deep breath, or a moment of gratitude , to celebrate.

Reflection: Ask yourself – How did breaking the goal into steps make it feel more achievable?

EVENING RITUAL – Wins and Worthiness

As night settles, reflect on your progress. Whether you completed one step or several, you've moved closer to your vision. Small steps create lasting change, and each one deserves acknowledgment.

Mantra: I honor flexibility and progress.

Action: In your *Confidence In Full Bloom Journal,* note one moment today when you successfully completed a step toward your goal.

Reflection: Ask yourself – How does acknowledging these small wins build confidence and trust in myself?

CLOSING THOUGHT:

Today, you nurtured your self-efficacy by breaking your SMART goal into smaller, doable steps. You owned your progress, honored your flexibility, and celebrated your wins. Each completed action is proof that growth is happening , one small, sacred step at a time.

Tomorrow, you'll take your SMART goal one step further by rooting it in time. When dreams move from "someday" to a set season, growth becomes not just possible , but inevitable.

DAY 6 – ROOTING SELF-EFFICACY: TIME-BOUND GROWTH

"Momentum blooms when intention meets time. The moment you honor your hours, your hours begin to honor you."

Namaste (Hindi), Magnificent Bloomer. You've planted your SMART goal, broken it into smaller steps, and learned to nurture each one with care. Today, you give your goals deeper roots by anchoring them in time. When you attach clear timelines to your actions, you transform your intention into motion and your motion into momentum. Each moment spent purposefully reinforces your self-trust and builds the steady rhythm that sustains growth.

MORNING RITUAL – Goals and Resourcefulness

Begin your morning with your Bloom Essentials , sip your Recharge Herbal Tea, stretch through your Rise Yoga Sequence, and breathe in your Resilient Essential Oils Blend. Let your body and mind awaken to the gentle promise of the day ahead. Then, focus on your SMART goal and decide when, exactly, you'll act. Time adds structure to your intention and invites your progress to take shape.

Mantra: Time-bound action creates momentum.

Action: Set time limits for one or more of your smaller SMART goal tasks. Be realistic but intentional.

Reflection: Ask yourself – What tools or strategies can help me stay on schedule and focused today?

Example of adding time limits:

If your SMART goal was to cook one healthy dinner at home three times this week, you might say:

- Pick out recipes by **12:00 p.m. today**.
- Write your grocery list by **12:30 p.m.**
- Shop by **6:30 p.m. tomorrow.**

By assigning time, you turn vague plans into specific commitments, and that's how confidence takes root.

MIDDAY RITUAL – Ownership and Alignment

At midday, pause for a quick recharge. Try a *Bloom Booster* to refocus your energy, deep breathing, a stretch, or a short walk outside. Then, return to your scheduled task with renewed clarity. Tracking what you do within time helps you take ownership of your choices and deepens your sense of self-leadership.

Mantra: I own my schedule and my effort.

Action: Complete at least one of your timed activities today and record how long it took in your *Confidence In Full Bloom Journal.*

Reflection: Ask yourself – How does claiming responsibility for my use of time affect my focus and energy?

EVENING RITUAL – Honoring Progress

As night settles, take a moment to honor your relationship with time. Whether you met your exact deadline or simply showed up with effort, you practiced presence and accountability. That is growth.

Mantra: I celebrate my punctual progress.

Action: Record the time you completed your activity in your journal and give yourself kudos for showing up intentionally.

Reflection: Ask yourself – What does honoring time teach me about trust, discipline, and self-efficacy?

CLOSING THOUGHT:

Today, you rooted your growth in time-bound intention. Each hour you shaped with purpose became an act of self-leadership, strengthening your confidence and your flow. Remember, Magnificent Bloomer: time is not your enemy, it's your ally. When you honor it, it carries your growth forward with grace and steady power.

DAY 7 – PLANTING SELF-EFFICACY: BIG FAT BLOOMING GOALS (BFBGs)

"Boldness is the sunlight of growth; it coaxes your hidden potential to rise and bloom."

Willkommen (German), Wonderful Bloomer. Today, you plant your first Big Fat Blooming Goal (BFBG) , a long-term, transformational vision designed to stretch and strengthen you over the next six to twelve months. Think of it as a *grand garden project* for your life , something that reshapes not only your habits but also your confidence and sense of purpose.

BFBGs are more than achievements; they're journeys of becoming. Each one calls you to grow beyond what's familiar, inviting courage, consistency, and belief. For physical wellness, that might mean training for a 5K, building strength through regular movement, mastering a new yoga practice, improving your sleep, or cultivating daily mindfulness and vitality. Whatever your BFBG may be, it should excite you, challenge you, and promise transformation.

MORNING RITUAL – Goals and Resourcefulness

Begin your day with your Bloom Essentials , sip your Recharge Herbal Tea, stretch through your Rise Yoga Sequence, and breathe in your Resilient Essential Oils Blend. As your body awakens, let your imagination expand toward possibility. Picture your life six months from now , stronger, lighter, more at peace. This is where your BFBG begins.

Mantra: I dream boldly and take action.

Action: Identify one *Big Fat Blooming Goal* for your physical wellness (or another area that calls to you) that you can realistically pursue over the next six to twelve months. Write it as a SMART goal in your *Confidence In Full Bloom Journal.*

Reflection: Ask yourself – Which resources, supports, and tools can help me pursue this goal over the coming months? How might achieving it transform my daily life and overall well-being?

Example BFBG:

I will train to run a 5K in under 35 minutes within 12 months by running three times per week, gradually increasing my distance and pace, and tracking my progress in my journal, so that I can complete the 5K and strengthen my cardiovascular fitness by [Month/Date].

MIDDAY RITUAL – Ownership and Courage

Pause midday and notice the pride that comes with taking ownership of a bold, long-term goal. Big dreams become real when you ground them in consistent, compassionate action. Even one small step forward today is enough to begin the journey.

Mantra: I own the power of my bold goal.

Action: Take one concrete step toward your BFBG. You might plan your workout schedule, prep your equipment, research a training guide, or set reminders to build a supportive daily habit. Pair your progress with a Physical Wellness *Bloom Booster* , a nourishing snack, a stretch, or a walk in fresh air , to keep your energy steady.

Reflection: Ask yourself – How does committing to this first step make me feel capable, energized, and ready for what's ahead?

EVENING RITUAL – Honoring Vision and Courage

As the day draws to a close, reflect on the courage it takes to dream beyond comfort and to begin something that matters deeply to you. Recognize your willingness to envision a greater version of yourself , that's how transformation starts.

Mantra: I celebrate daring to dream.

Action: In your *Confidence In Full Bloom Journal,* record the first step you took toward your BFBG today and how it felt to take action.

Reflection: Ask yourself – How does envisioning and beginning this goal strengthen my belief in my own courage and capacity for change?

CLOSING THOUGHT:

Today, you planted the seed of a bold, beautiful goal , one that will stretch your confidence and expand your life. Through imagination, ownership, and celebration, you've proven that you can dream with direction and act with purpose. Each small step from this point forward will water your courage and cultivate your confidence.

Tomorrow, you'll begin watering your *Big Fat Blooming Goal* with **Bloom Steps** and **Root Steps** , smaller, intentional actions that keep your dream alive, even on the busiest days. Just like a flourishing garden, your BFBG will grow with steady care, patience, and love.

DAY 8 – WATERING SELF-EFFICACY: BLOOM AND ROOT STEPS

"Big dreams grow strong when watered by small, faithful actions."

Ciao (Italian), Charming Bloomer. Today, you nurture the bold goal you planted yesterday , your Big Fat Blooming Goal (BFBG). Remember, transformation doesn't happen all at once; it unfolds through steady, intentional care. Big goals flourish when they're supported by small, consistent steps , the kind you can see, feel, and celebrate along the way.

To keep your momentum alive, you'll learn to pair your actions into two types of steps:

- **Bloom Steps** , the *direct actions* that move you forward. These are the moments of doing: jogging for five minutes, completing a yoga sequence, writing a page, or recording your first video.
- **Root Steps** , the *supportive actions* that prepare you for success. These might be setting out your workout clothes, queuing up your yoga playlist, clearing your workspace, or setting a timer to protect your focus.

When Bloom Steps and Root Steps work together, progress feels steady, sustainable, and grounded. Roots nourish blooms , and blooms remind you why the roots matter.

MORNING RITUAL – Goals and Resourcefulness

Begin your morning with your Bloom Essentials , sip your Recharge Herbal Tea, stretch through your Rise Yoga Sequence, and breathe in your Resilient Essential Oils Blend. Let your breath and movement remind you that progress begins with presence. Then, turn to your BFBG and make it tangible.

Mantra: Big goals grow with small, consistent steps.

Action: Identify at least one *Bloom Step* and one *Root Step* for your BFBG. For example, if your BFBG is completing a 5K, your Bloom Step might be jogging for five minutes, while your Root Step could be setting out your running clothes the night before.

Reflection: Ask yourself – How does breaking my goal into paired steps make it feel more real and achievable?

MIDDAY RITUAL – Ownership and Mapping Progress

Pause midday and take time to organize your ideas into a visual plan. Open your *Confidence In Full Bloom Journal* or use a simple two-column list , one side for Bloom Steps, one for Root Steps. This pairing helps you see how preparation and action rely on one another.

Mantra: I take ownership of progress in motion.

Action: Write at least three *Bloom–Root Step* pairs for your BFBG in your journal or notebook. For example, if your BFBG is to master a yoga sequence, your Bloom Step might be completing a flow, and your Root Step could be creating a quiet space and cueing your playlist.

Reflection: Ask yourself – How does seeing my steps organized on paper make the goal feel achievable and clear? Which steps spark the most motivation or joy?

EVENING RITUAL – Clarity and Confidence

As evening approaches, take a moment to reflect on how your planning shaped your sense of direction. Clarity itself is progress. Each paired step you identified today strengthens your self-efficacy , showing you that your dream is not only possible but already in motion.

Mantra: I celebrate incremental growth.

Action: In your journal, record one insight about your task breakdown. Note which Bloom–Root pair feels most doable for tomorrow and why.

Reflection: Ask yourself – How does today's organization and reflection reinforce my confidence? How does mapping my steps ease overwhelm and increase readiness?

CLOSING THOUGHT:

Today, you watered your bold goal by breaking it into Bloom and Root Steps , small, mindful actions that transform big visions into daily movement. You've given your dream structure, rhythm, and life. Each Bloom–Root pairing is a promise: that you can stay grounded while reaching higher.

Tomorrow, you'll deepen your growth by adding **time, sequence, and tracking** to your steps , turning your BFBG into a living rhythm of progress. With each intentional move, your garden of goals grows stronger, steadier, and more radiant.

DAY 9 – ROOTING SELF-EFFICACY: BRINGING YOUR BFBG TO LIFE

"Time gives dreams structure, and structure gives them breath."

Salutations (Latin org.), Sensational Bloomer. Yesterday, you gave shape to your Big Fat Blooming Goal (BFBG) by identifying your Bloom–Root Step pairs , those small, powerful actions that turn big dreams into daily movement. Today, you'll root those steps in *time* by scheduling, sequencing, and tracking them. This is the moment your bold goal shifts from an inspiring idea to a living, breathing plan.

When you give your steps a home in time, you transform potential into progress. When you sequence them, you create a natural rhythm of action. When you track them, you build accountability and self-trust. Together, these practices help you stay grounded in your purpose and motivated by your progress.

MORNING RITUAL – Goals and Resourcefulness

Begin your day with your **Bloom Essentials** , sip your *Recharge Herbal Tea*, stretch through your *Rise Yoga Sequence*, and breathe in your *Resilient Essential Oils Blend*. Let these rituals remind you that time is a sacred resource , one you can shape intentionally.

Mantra: A goal with time becomes a living path.

Action: Choose one Bloom Step from your BFBG and assign it a specific time today. For example, if your BFBG is running a 5K, commit to a 10-minute jog at 7:00 a.m. or 6:00 p.m. Record it in your planner, journal, or calendar.

Reflection: Ask yourself – How does putting my action into time make it feel more real and possible?

MIDDAY RITUAL – Ownership and Structure

As the day unfolds, deepen your ownership by creating sequence and structure. Open your *Confidence In Full Bloom Journal* or use a simple spreadsheet or notebook. Arrange your Bloom–Root Step pairs in the order they must happen and assign time frames for each. Then, choose a tracking method that supports you , a journal entry, a checklist, a habit tracker, smart phone notes, or even a sticky note on your mirror.

Mantra: I create structure that supports my success.

Action: List at least three Bloom–Root Step pairs, organize them in sequence, and assign realistic time frames. For instance, if your BFBG is building strength, your plan might look like this:

- **Bloom Step:** Two workouts per week (Months 1–2) → three workouts per week (Months 3–5) → complete a challenge (Months 6–8).
- **Root Steps:** Schedule gym time, prepare workout gear, log progress in an app.
- **Reflection:** Ask yourself – How does sequencing my steps and choosing a tracking method help me feel more capable and prepared? Which tracking method feels natural and motivating to me?

EVENING RITUAL – Wins and Reflection

As night falls, take a moment to celebrate your transformation from dreamer to doer. You've turned your bold idea into a grounded, time-bound plan. Every step scheduled, every sequence written, every system chosen is a promise to your future self.

Mantra: I celebrate my progress becoming visible.

Action: Record one timed Bloom Step you completed today and note how you'll track tomorrow's next action.

Reflection: Ask yourself – How does giving my goal structure ease my mind and build my motivation? How does having a clear plan strengthen my trust in my ability to follow through?

CLOSING THOUGHT:

Today, you rooted your BFBG in the fertile ground of time, structure, and accountability. Your goal now lives on your schedule , not just in your imagination. You've taken the brave leap from vision to motion, and that deserves deep recognition.

Tomorrow, we'll honor *consistency* , the quiet rhythm that sustains growth. Some days, you'll cross off several steps; other days, the victory will simply be showing up and doing one small thing to keep your dream alive. If you didn't finish today, take a breath. That's okay. Progress is not perfection , it's persistence.

Remember, Beautiful Bloomer: your confidence grows each time you choose to keep going.

DAY 10 – BLOOMING SELF-EFFICACY CELEBRATION

"Growth is not measured by how fast you move, but by how faithfully you keep showing up."

Marhaba (Arabic) Marvelous Bloomer. You've reached a milestone worth celebrating. Over the past ten days, you've planted seeds of confidence, nurtured consistency, created SMART goals, and dared to name a Big Fat Blooming Goal (BFBG) that stretches your potential. You've shown yourself what steady effort and self-trust can do.

Today is about reflection and celebration, not perfection. Whether your BFBG is still in planning or already sprouting progress, this moment is your reminder that growth is a journey of becoming. You've cultivated self-efficacy , the belief in your ability to take action and create results , and that belief is now rooted within you.

MORNING RITUAL – Gratitude and Reflection

Begin your day with your **Bloom Essentials**, sip your *Recharge Herbal Tea*, stretch gently through your *Rise Yoga Sequence*, and breathe deeply with your *Resilient Essential Oils Blend*. Let this be a soft exhale of gratitude for all you've accomplished.

Mantra: I thrive in effort and results.

Action: Reflect on all the goals and milestones you've achieved during this phase. Choose one joyful way to celebrate your effort , a walk outside, dancing to your favorite song, or savoring a nourishing meal.

Reflection: Ask yourself – Which habits, supports, or moments of courage helped me grow the most?

MIDDAY RITUAL – Ownership and Pride

At midday, take a pause to honor your ownership of this journey. You've shown up , even on the days when it felt easier not to. Your consistency has turned intention into evidence.

Mantra: I own my journey fully.

Action: Share your wins out loud , with a friend, a loved one, or simply in your journal. Read back through your entries from the past ten days and notice how your tone, clarity, and confidence have evolved.

Reflection: Ask yourself – How does acknowledging my growth strengthen my belief in what's possible next?

EVENING RITUAL – Celebration and Renewal

As dusk settles, close this phase with celebration and serenity. You've built something beautiful inside yourself , a quiet confidence that will continue to bloom.

Mantra: I celebrate my unstoppable growth.

Action: End the day with a joyful wellness ritual , dance freely, soak in a calming bath, or unwind with restorative yoga. Let every movement say, *"I did this. I am proud."*

Reflection: Ask yourself – How does celebrating my effort and progress make me feel in my body and spirit?

CLOSING THOUGHT:

Today you've honored your effort, your consistency, and your courage. You've proven to yourself that growth is possible , one small, intentional act at a time.

Your self-efficacy now lives in motion, not just in theory. It's in every time you tried again, adjusted your plan, or kept going when no one was watching. Remember: your BFBG doesn't have to be finished , it just has to be *alive*.

Take your time, trust your rhythm, and know this; your ability to follow through is the bloom itself. You are becoming everything you believed you could be.

PHASE 2 – SELF-EFFICACY: CLOSING SUMMARY

Congratulations, Bold Bloomer. You've just completed the ten-day journey of *self-efficacy*, a season of steady, embodied growth. Over these past days, you have proven that confidence isn't something we wait to feel; it's something we *build* through small, intentional acts of follow-through.

You began by planting simple goals, tiny seeds of belief that reminded you, "I can." From there, you nurtured SMART goals, structured steps that turned intention into action. And finally, you dared to dream beyond the ordinary by naming your *Big Fat Blooming Goal (BFBG)*your bold vision for transformation. Each stage has rooted your confidence deeper and helped your self-trust rise taller.

This phase followed the **GROW** Bloomprint cadence:

- **Morning – Goals and Resourcefulness:** You started each day by setting clear intentions, identifying your supports, and preparing your mind and body to act.
- **Midday – Ownership:** You took responsibility for your actions, held yourself accountable, and practiced persistence even when energy wavered.
- **Evening – Wins:** You reflected on progress, honored small victories, and recognized that every completed step, no matter how modest, was evidence of your capability.

Your *Bloom At-Home Physical Wellness Practices* guided this journey: mindful movement, consistent journaling, small acts of accountability, and intentional celebration. Each repetition deepened your self-discipline, expanded your self-belief, and revealed that growth doesn't demand perfection, only presence.

- Through these practices, you've learned to:
- Start small, stay consistent, and grow steadily.
- Use structure (SMART goals) to create freedom.
- Dream boldly, then bring those dreams to life through actionable steps.
- Trust that progress, not perfection, is what builds lasting confidence.

This phase has shown that **self-efficacy is a muscle**, one strengthened by clarity, commitment, and compassion. Every time you kept a promise to yourself, you rewired your belief that you *can.*

Carry forward the rhythm of **GROW:**

- Set your Goals with intention.
- Recognize your Resources.
- Own your actions fully.
- Celebrate your WINs daily.

Each cycle builds momentum. Each win, no matter how small, prepares you to rise higher in your wellness and your life.

You've completed the second leg of your *My Life In Full Bloom* journey, and that's no small thing. You've proven to yourself that you can trust your follow-through. Take a deep breath, smile, and feel the pride of that truth settling in your bones.

When you're ready, complete your **Post-Blooming Self-Efficacy Quick Assessment** to see how your confidence and capability have expanded after ten days of practicing and building physical wellness.

Post – Blooming Self-Efficacy Quick Assessment

Instructions: For each statement, rate yourself from **1 (Not at all true)** to **5 (Completely true).** Tally your score at the end and compare to Day 0.

Part 1: Quick Self-Check

		1-5
1	I celebrate small victories along the way.	
2	I stay motivated to continue my wellness practices.	
3	I feel a sense of accomplishment from wellness actions.	
4	I feel confident in my ability to reach my goals.	
5	I trust myself to take consistent action.	
6	I can handle challenges and adapt when needed.	
7	I set and track physical or wellness goals regularly.	
8	I take deliberate action to care for my wellness.	
9	I use available resources to help me succeed.	
	Total	

Part 2: Blooming Reflections:

What shifted most for me over the last 10 days?

Which practice(s) felt the most empowering for me?

Part 3: My Victory Statement
In your journal, write a short declaration that celebrates your blooming.

Post Physical Wellness Check-in: Shade and name the pie. Then review Day 1.

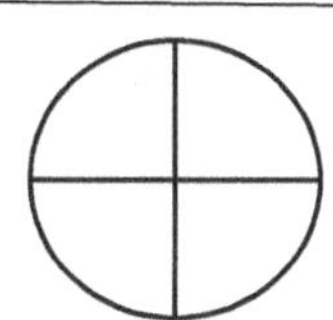

My current state:

Blooming Reflection: The Courage to Keep Growing

> Pause for a moment, Lovely Bloomer.
>
> Look at all you've accomplished. You've set goals, kept promises to yourself, and discovered that self-efficacy grows not through perfection, but through steady, intentional effort.
>
> You are becoming your own evidence of what's possible.
>
> Every step , big or small, has built trust in your ability to make things happen.
>
> If you need a break, take it.
>
> This is your journey, unfolding in your time. You are allowed to rest, reassess, and return whenever you're ready.
>
> What matters most is that you don't stop moving forward. Keep nurturing your goals with kindness and curiosity.
>
> You've proven that you can show up for yourself; again, and again.
>
> Next, in Phase 3: Self-Love, you'll deepen that trust.
>
> Together, we'll turn all your effort into tenderness, learning to love the woman who made it this far.
>
> Because she's worth every bit of care, every single day.

Phase 3:

Blooming Self-Love

Welcome to Self-Love. This is where your journey of embracing and celebrating yourself fully blooms. Self-love is the sunlight that nourishes and energizes everything else, compassion, joy, and true acceptance of who you are.

Anchor List for Phase 3

1. Take Your Self-Love & Spiritual Wellness Assessments - Awareness is the first act of confidence

2. Create Your BYO Bloom-At-Home Well-ness Plan- Choose rituals and rhythms that help you feel grounded and nourished each day.

3. Meet Celine - Your Phase 3 story companion.

4. Practice Self-Love for the next ten days.

Blooming Self-Love Quick Assessments

SELF-LOVE ASSESSMENT

Instructions: For each statement, rate yourself from **1 (Not at all true)** to **5 (Completely true).** Total your points at the end.

Part 1: Inner Acceptance

		1-5
1	I feel a sense of self-love and acceptance.	
2	I honor my inner voice and feelings.	
3	I feel aligned with my purpose and values.	

Part 2: Daily Care and Joy

		1-5
4	I practice daily rituals or habits that nourish my mind, body, and spirit.	
5	I make time for activities that bring me joy.	
6	I notice my growth and celebrate my wins.	
7	I feel optimistic and ready to manifest positive change in my life.	

Part 3: Relationships and Compassion

		1-5
8	I connect meaningfully with others and share positive energy.	
9	I perform acts of kindness or compassion for others.	

Total ☐

See the Self-Love assessment key on the next page. Then, complete the Spiritual Wellness Check and set a goal for the next 10 days.

Blooming Self-Love Quick Assessment – Key

- **9–18:** Your self-love garden is ready for planting. This phase will help you nurture new roots of compassion and acceptance.
- **19–31:** You have some blooming buds of self-love. Over the next 10 days, you'll strengthen and expand them.
- **32–45**: You radiate a keen sense of self-love. Use this phase to deepen, sustain, and celebrate your flourishing.

SPIRITUAL WELLNESS CHECK AND GOAL SETTING

This visual reflection helps you assess your current spiritual wellness and set heartfelt intentions for growth during your **Self-Love phase**. You'll return to this same page on **Day 10** to reflect on your healing and progress.

What This Measures

Your spiritual wellness pie represents your connection to love, meaning, and inner peace, especially your ability to extend compassion toward yourself and others. Consider:

- How connected you feel to something greater than yourself (love, faith, nature, community, Source)
- Whether you find meaning or wisdom in life's challenges
- How your values and beliefs nurture self-compassion and forgiveness

Instructions

Step 1: Measure Your Current Wellness: Look at the pie chart divided into four quarters (each worth 25% for a total of 100%). Using a colored pencil, crayon, or marker, shade in the amount that represents your spiritual wellness TODAY.

____

My current state:

Shading Guide:

- **4 full quarters (100%)** – You feel deeply grounded in love, peace, and purpose.
- **3 full quarters (75%)** – You feel spiritually connected but still have moments of doubt or disconnection.
- **2 full quarters (50%)** – You're rebuilding trust in yourself and your beliefs after emotional setbacks.
- **1 full quarter (25%)** – You're struggling to reconnect with hope or self-compassion.
- **No shading (0%)** – You feel spiritually lost or cut off from love, faith, or meaning.
- **Partial quarters:** Shade portions of a quarter for more precise percentages.

Example: If your spiritual wellness feels around 62%, shade two full quarters (50%) and half of the third quarter (12%).

Step 2: Name Your Current State: On the line above your shaded pie, write a name that captures spiritual condition right now.

Examples of naming:

- "Learning to Love Myself Through It All"
- "Faith in Progress"
- "Reconnecting with My Inner Light"
- "Rooted in Grace, Still Healing"

Step 3: Explain Current State: Next to your pie, write 2-3 sentences describing:

- Points of connection: Where do you feel spiritually strong or supported? What gives you peace or purpose?
- Points of questioning: What feels uncertain or distant? How has self-doubt or pain affected your faith or trust in yourself?

Example: "I feel grounded when I meditate or spend quiet time in nature, it helps me remember I'm part of something bigger (connection). But I still struggle to fully forgive myself for past mistakes and to believe that I deserve unconditional love (questioning)."

Step 4: Set Your 10-Day Goal

In the space provided, shade a second pie showing where you hope your **spiritual wellness** will be after ten days of practicing self-love.

I hope to improve my physical wellness by..."

Step 5: Write Your Intention

Complete this sentence: "Over the next 10 days, I hope to improve my spiritual wellness by..."

Examples:

- "...reconnecting with quiet rituals that remind me I am loved and supported."
- "...forgiving myself for not being perfect and trusting that I'm growing through grace."
- "...spending time in reflection or prayer to rebuild trust in my own heart."
- "...finding stillness each day to listen to the gentle voice within that says, 'You are enough.'"

This becomes your visual target for the next ten days, your reminder that peace grows through presence and care.

BYO Bloom At-Home Spiritual Wellness Plan

This is your moment to design a wellness plan that speaks to your soul. See Appendices B: 3a and B:3b. Choose the Bloom At-Home Wellness practices that call to you. What helps you feel grounded, peaceful, safe, and whole? There's no right or wrong. Let your heart and health lead you. Use the space below to build you plan:

Plan 1

Sunrise	
Midday	
Bedtime	

Plan 2

Sunrise	
Midday	
Bedtime	

Plan 3

Sunrise	
Midday	
Bedtime	

CELINE'S STORY: Learning to Love Herself Forward

Celine didn't see the layoff coming. One Thursday morning, she was leading a project meeting over Teams; by that afternoon, she was boxing up her things under the dull hum of an office that suddenly felt too quiet, too cold.

Six years of loyalty, late nights, and bright ideas that rarely carried her name, and now she was just another name on a spreadsheet.

For a while, she moved through her days in a fog. Anger. Numbness. Endless scrolling through job boards, rewriting résumés that no human might ever read. She told herself she just needed "a fresh start," but deep down, she knew what she really needed was to stop *starting over* for everyone but herself.

What she didn't know yet was that her healing wouldn't come from a new position, or a paycheck. It would come from something smaller. Quieter. Softer.

One Saturday morning, her daughter Leila woke up crying with another eczema flare-up. Celine felt helpless. But then, she remembered her grandmother's old olive oil soap, the way the house used to smell of lavender and summer evenings, how her grandmother's hands looked so sure, stirring healing into every batch.

So, she decided to try. She found a recipe online, mixed a few oils she had on hand, and made a small batch in her kitchen. Olive oil. Shea butter. A drop of lavender. Simple. Unassuming. But when her kids' skin began to heal, something inside her did too.

It started as soap. But it became something sacred; something that said, *You still have magic in you.*

She began sharing the bars with friends. Then friends of friends. They loved the scent, the story, the heart in it. One day, a neighbor said, "You should sell this." And for the first time in a long while, Celine didn't laugh it off.

Instead of saying, "Who am I to do that?" She asked, "Why not me?"

She taught herself to design her own labels, photograph her products, write her brand story, even to use AI tools to help her grow. With each new skill, she wasn't just learning business, she was learning herself.

Soon, *Ah-live*, her small-batch soap line, was born. But more than a business, it became a love letter, to her children, her grandmother, her community, and the woman she was finally learning to love.

Her evenings began to look different. The glow of the TV was replaced with candlelight and the scent of lavender. Her hands moved with intention again. And in that rhythm, she began to remember who she was before the world told her she had to prove it.

The biggest change wasn't in her career; it was in her conversation with herself. She stopped saying, *"I'm not enough."* And started saying, *"I'm becoming," Michele Obama style,*

Celine gave herself permission to try, to fail, to rest, to rise. And in that permission, she found a love that didn't need to be earned, it just needed to be remembered.

Nurturing Self-Love the Celine Way

Celine's story reminds us that self-love doesn't arrive as lightning; it grows quietly, like a seed that's been waiting for sunlight.

It begins the moment you decide to care for yourself, even when you don't feel worthy yet.

It deepens when you create something that nourishes you, in a world that often profits from your depletion.

It expands every time you say, I am allowed to start over, for me this time.

By trusting her creativity and letting technology become a tool, not a threat, Celine turned her fear into fuel.

Her self-love didn't appear all at once, it emerged gently, like the soft lather in her hands, through patience, practice, and grace.

Celine's story is a love note to every woman learning to love herself forward:

When the system no longer serves you, build something that does.

When the noise outside gets too loud, listen to the quiet inside.

And when doubt whispers, "*Who do you think you are?*" Whisper back, " *I'm becoming who I was always meant to be.*"

Self-love is not about perfection. It's about permission; the permission to bloom, right here, right now, in the middle of your own becoming.

And, as everyone knows, to say a woman is "becoming," is to call her beautiful!

Blooming Self – Love: Daily Practice

"Love is the sunlight that calls every hidden part of you to rise."

Radiant Bloomer, these final ten days are your season of soft expansion , a time to honor how far you've come and to love yourself, fully, in motion. You'll move through the **BLOOM** cadence each day ; Balance, Love, Open-heartedness, Optimism, and Manifestation, gentle practices that help you live your wholeness out loud.

Morning (B & L): Begin with your Bloom Essentials , sip your Restore Tea Blend, flow through your Release Yoga Sequence, and breathe in your Radiance Essential Oil Blend from Appendix B:3a. Feel balance return to your body, then meet your reflection with love. Whisper something kind to yourself before the day begins.

Midday (O & O): Open your heart to joy. Choose a Bloom Booster from your BYO or Appendix B:3b , dance, laugh, share a kindness, or savor something beautiful. Let optimism infuse your afternoon like sunlight through glass.

Evening (M): Manifest peace. Reflect on the moments you loved yourself well today, and name one intention for tomorrow's growth.

Keep your Confidence in Full Bloom Journal, pen, and Bloom Essentials nearby.

Each time you cycle through BLOOM, you return to your natural state , balanced, brave, and beautifully alive.

DAY 1: PLANTING SEEDS OF GRATITUDE & PRESENCE

"Love begins with attention to your breath, your being, this very moment."

As-salaamu alaykum (Egyptian), Alluring Bloomer. Today you begin the third phase of your journey: Self-Love , the art of being fully awake to yourself and the moment you're in. Presence is not about perfection; it's about noticing what *is* , your breath, your sensations, your emotions , and choosing to meet them with tenderness. Gratitude deepens this awareness, reminding you that even now, there is so much to love and appreciate.

When you anchor yourself in gratitude, you stop chasing what's missing and start blooming from what's already here , your strength, your softness, your becoming.

MORNING RITUAL – Balance and Love

Begin with your Bloom Essentials , sip your Restore Tea Blend, flow through your Release Yoga Sequence, and breathe in your Radiance Essential Oil Blend. Feel balance return to your body, then meet your reflection with love.

Mantra: I am present, and I honor myself with gratitude.

Action: In your *Confidence In Full Bloom Journal*, write one observation from your mind, one from your body, and one from your spirit. Add one thing you are grateful for in each.

Reflection: Ask yourself – How does gratitude shift the way I experience my needs and my presence today?

MIDDAY RITUAL – Open-heartedness

Pause in the middle of your day and open your heart to joy. Choose a Bloom Booster , mindful breathing, a gratitude walk or simply noticing beauty in something small.

Mantra: Gratitude opens my heart to joy.

Action: Name three things you are grateful for right now and allow yourself to feel each one fully.

Reflection: Ask yourself – How did practicing gratitude shift my connection to myself and others today?

EVENING RITUAL – Manifesting Peace

As evening settles, return to stillness. Reflect on how presence and gratitude have carried you through the day.

Mantra: I rest in gratitude for what is and trust in what is becoming.

Action: In your journal, list three moments from today that you are most grateful for.

Reflection: Ask yourself – How does ending my day in gratitude nurture peace, optimism, and self-love?

CLOSING THOUGHT:

Today you planted the first seeds of self-love through presence and gratitude. By honoring this moment and cherishing what already exists within you, you've created fertile soil for deeper love to grow. Rest knowing that you are already blooming , just by being here, aware, and beautifully you.

DAY 2 – PREPARING THE SOUL

"Before love blooms, it takes root in what we dare to imagine."

Jambo (Swahili), Joyful Bloomer. Today, you plant the seed of **vision**, the sacred art of seeing yourself whole, thriving, and aligned with love. Vision is not fantasy; it's faith with form. It's how you begin to shape the life your spirit already knows you're worthy of living. When you see your future self, radiant, grounded, and joyful, you prepare your inner soil to receive it.

MORNING RITUAL – Balance and Love

Begin with your Self-Love Bloom Essentials , sip your Restore Tea Blend, flow through your Release Yoga Sequence, and breathe in your Radiance Essential Oil Blend. Let presence settle you into balance.

Mantra: I am whole and grounded in love.

Action: In your *Confidence In Full Bloom Journal,* write one observation from your mind, body, and spirit. Then, respond lovingly to each, what does each part need today?

Reflection: Ask yourself – How does noticing and responding to my needs help me feel cared for and supported?

MIDDAY RITUAL – Open-heartedness

Vision grows in open hearts. Pause and practice a Spiritual Wellness Bloom Booster, perhaps a short meditation or a moment of mindful breathing. Picture your future self already living in love.

Mantra: I open my heart to joy and possibility.

Action: Take five minutes to visualize your future self, radiant, calm, and free.

Reflection: Ask yourself – How did connecting with my future self expand my sense of possibility and joy?

EVENING RITUAL – Optimism and Manifestation

As night falls, bring your awareness to your unfolding journey. Every dream begins in your imagination, believe in its becoming.

Mantra: I hold a loving vision for my future.

Action: Write one loving affirmation that reflects your vision of self-love, something you wish to live into.

Reflection: Ask yourself – How does visualizing my future self in love change how I show up for myself tonight?

CLOSING THOUGHT:

Today you prepared the soul of your self-love journey by planting vision, your compass for what's to come. Each time you return to this vision with love, you remind yourself that you are both the dream and the dreamer. Tomorrow, you'll plant the seed of commitment, where love turns from wishful to powerful, one promise, one act, one moment at a time.

DAY 3: PLANTING THE SEED OF COMMITMENT

"Commitment is love in motion , the daily promise to keep showing up for yourself."

Nǐ hǎo (Chinese), Insightful Bloomer. Today, you plant the seed of commitment , the sacred rhythm that transforms intention into transformation. Commitment isn't about striving for perfection; it's about presence. It's the quiet agreement between your heart and your higher self to keep showing up, even when it's hard, even when it's quiet. Like a steady heartbeat, your commitment keeps your self-love alive and growing.

MORNING RITUAL – Balance and Love

Begin with your Self-Love Bloom Essentials , sip your Restore Tea Blend, flow through your Release Yoga Sequence, and breathe in your Radiance Essential Oil Blend. Feel yourself arrive in this moment. Presence is your first act of devotion.

Mantra: I commit to showing up for myself with love.

Action: Spend ten minutes in mindful presence , journaling, meditating, or gentle yoga. Choose a practice you can return to tomorrow.

Reflection: Ask yourself – What does it look like for me to keep showing up, even when it feels hard?

MIDDAY RITUAL – Open-heartedness

Commitment doesn't have to feel heavy; it can hum with joy. When you infuse your promises with pleasure, you make showing up something to look forward to.

Mantra: I find joy in the promises I keep to myself.

Action: Practice your joyful ritual , perhaps a mindful walk, a favorite song, or a laughter break. Let joy become part of your discipline.

Reflection: Ask yourself – How did keeping this joyful promise to myself shift my energy today?

EVENING RITUAL – Optimism and Manifestation

As evening settles, let gratitude anchor your growth. Trust that your steady care is shaping something beautiful within you.

Mantra: I trust the process of my steady growth.

Action: Write three commitments you honored today, no matter how small, and one you'll carry into tomorrow.

Reflection: Ask yourself – How does gratitude for today's commitments help me trust my growth tomorrow?

CLOSING THOUGHT:

Today, you planted the seed of commitment , your steady devotion to self-love. Each promise kept becomes a root of confidence and compassion. Remember, commitment is not about doing more; it's about returning to what matters most , you. Tomorrow, you'll replenish your spirit by learning how to refill your cup so love can flow through you freely, like rain nourishing the earth.

DAY 4: WATERING SELF-LOVE

"Self-love, like any living thing, needs steady nourishment, care given not once, but again and again."

Sawasdee ka (Thai), Spectacular Bloomer. Today, you turn your attention to watering the seeds of self-love you've planted. In nature, watering keeps a seed alive long enough to reach the light. In your life, watering means tending to your spirit through compassion, care, and daily attention. Without this steady flow of kindness, even the strongest intentions can wither.

Watering is a practice of presence, choosing to notice your needs and responding with gentleness. It's about giving yourself permission to receive what you give so freely to others. Each act of care, no matter how small, nourishes your roots and prepares your heart to bloom.

MORNING RITUAL – Balance and Love

Begin your morning with your Self-Love Bloom Essentials , sip your Restore Tea Blend, flow through your Release Yoga Sequence, and breathe in your Radiance Essential Oil Blend. Let calm energy wash through you. Treat yourself as you would a cherished friend: tenderly, without judgment.

Mantra: I am kind to myself and my needs.

Action: Stand before a mirror, place your hand over your heart, and say aloud three times: *"I am worthy of love and care."* Feel the words settle deep within you.

Reflection: Ask yourself – How does practicing compassion shift how I feel about myself right now?

MIDDAY RITUAL – Open-heartedness

Love expands when you share it. Just as rain nourishes an entire garden, your kindness can refresh another's spirit while replenishing your own.

Mantra: I open to connection and sacred joy.

Action: Reach out to someone you appreciate. Send a short note, a kind message, or a moment of gratitude. Notice how giving love creates space for more within you.

Reflection: Ask yourself – How did extending love to another elevate my own joy and sense of belonging?

EVENING RITUAL – Optimism and Manifestation

As the day softens, water your dreams with hope. Visualization keeps your future in bloom by helping you see what's already possible.

Mantra: I see the light in my future.

Action: Close your eyes and picture yourself thriving , calm, confident, and radiant. Let that image take root in your heart.

Reflection: Ask yourself – How does seeing myself thriving help me believe in the possibilities ahead?

CLOSING THOUGHT:

Today, you've watered your self-love with compassion, connection, and vision. Every drop of kindness, toward yourself or another, feeds your becoming. Keep tending these waters with care; the garden of your heart grows stronger with every act of love. Tomorrow, you'll deepen your roots by practicing grounding and renewal, building the quiet stability that allows every bloom to reach for the light.

DAY 5: GERMINATING SELF-LOVE

"Growth begins quietly; in the tender moment you choose to notice your own becoming."

Salut (French), Astute Bloomer. Today, you honor the early stirrings of your self-love. Germination is that sacred moment when a seed breaks open and reaches toward the light. Likewise, your spirit expands each time you offer yourself consistency, creativity, and care. Germination asks for patience , to trust the unseen work happening beneath the surface, knowing that each small act of love strengthens your roots and prepares you to bloom.

MORNING RITUAL – Balance and Love

Begin with your Self-Love Bloom Essentials , sip your Restore Tea Blend, flow through your Release Yoga Sequence, and breathe in your Radiance Essential Oil Blend. Let your morning unfold slowly, noticing your mind, body, and spirit with compassion. Awareness itself is an act of love.

Mantra: I honor my growth with balance and love.

Action: In your Confidence in Full Bloom Journal, note one observation from your mind, one from your body, and one from your spirit. Write a kind, supportive response to each.

Reflection: Ask yourself – What did I learn about myself by noticing with compassion?

MIDDAY RITUAL – Open-heartedness

Let your creativity and spirit breathe. Self-love grows when you give your inner world light through music, stillness, movement, or gratitude.

Mantra: I open my heart to creativity and light.

Action: Choose one Spiritual Wellness Bloom Booster , meditate, take a mindful walk, or write a gratitude list. Let it be simple and joyful.

Reflection: Ask yourself – How did this practice nourish my inner light and strengthen my sense of self-love?

EVENING RITUAL – Optimism and Manifestation

As dusk arrives, tend your growing self-love with hope. Optimism is the sunlight that guides new growth; manifestation is your trust in its unfolding.

Mantra: I am optimistic and aligned with purpose.

Action: In your Confidence in Full Bloom Journal, write one intention for tomorrow that supports your self-love , rest, play, patience, or creativity.

Reflection: Ask yourself – How does setting this intention energize me for what's to come?

CLOSING THOUGHT:

Today, you honored the gentle beginnings of your self-love through awareness, creativity, and purpose. These early sprouts of care remind you that even quiet growth is powerful. Trust the process , your bloom has already begun.

DAY 6: ROOTING IN SELF-LOVE

"Strength is not only in how high you rise, but in how deeply you are willing to root."

G'day (Australian) Clever Bloomer. Today, you anchor your self-love more deeply. Just as a flower's bloom depends on its roots, your spirit flourishes when you feel grounded in who you are. Rooting is about stability, honoring your needs, setting boundaries, and nurturing connections that support your growth. When your roots run deep, you can draw strength from your values, weather life's storms, and flourish with quiet confidence.

MORNING RITUAL – Balance and Love

Begin with your Self-Love Bloom Essentials , sip your Restore Tea Blend, flow through your Release Yoga Sequence, and breathe in your Radiance Essential Oil Blend. As you ground into presence, acknowledge your needs without judgment.

Mantra: I honor and nourish my whole self.

Action: In your Confidence in Full Bloom Journal, write one boundary or self-care need you will honor today , for example, "I will rest before saying yes" or "I will speak gently to myself."

Reflection: Ask yourself – How does naming and honoring this need strengthen my sense of self-love?

MIDDAY RITUAL – Open-heartedness

Extend your roots into connection. Like trees intertwining beneath the soil, our spirits are strengthened by community and kindness.

Mantra: I root myself in joy and community.

Action: Reach out to someone today , offer encouragement, gratitude, or a simple hello. Notice how giving and receiving care nourish you both.

Reflection: Ask yourself – How did this act of connection deepen my sense of belonging and support?

EVENING RITUAL – Optimism and Manifestation

As the day closes, align your heart with purpose. Rooting in optimism means trusting that your growth is supported by something steady and good.

Mantra: I root myself in purpose and possibility.

Action: In your Confidence in Full Bloom Journal, write one intention that anchors your self-love , perhaps, "I will trust myself more deeply" or "I will create peace through daily gratitude."

Reflection: Ask yourself – How does aligning with this intention make me feel more secure and strong?

CLOSING THOUGHT:

Today, you strengthened your foundation through self-honor, connection, and clarity of purpose. Each rooted choice nourishes your growth, giving you the stability to rise higher and bloom brighter. Tomorrow, you'll begin lifting your self-love into visibility , letting your light be seen, shared, and celebrated.

DAY 7: SPROUTING SELF-LOVE

"When the heart is ready, even the smallest light becomes an invitation to grow."

Oi (Brazilian), Breathtaking Bloomer. Today, your self-love begins to sprout, tender and green, reaching toward the light. What was once unseen within you now stirs, stretching past the quiet soil of reflection into the visible world. Sprouting is a sacred unveiling, the moment when self-love moves from thought into living, breathing form. It's how your care, your peace, and your courage begin to show up in how you move, speak, and see yourself. Be gentle with this newness. Every sprout is soft at first, but strength lives within its reach.

MORNING RITUAL – Balance and Love

Begin your morning with your Self-Love Bloom Essentials , sip your Restore Tea Blend, move through your Release Yoga Sequence, and breathe in your Radiance Essential Oil Blend. Let the calmness rise through you like morning light spreading across a quiet field. Peace is the ground where love takes root and sprouts toward the sun.

Mantra: I breathe peace into my becoming.

Action: Sit quietly for a few moments after your Bloom Essentials. Feel your breath. Notice how your heart softens as stillness enters. In your Confidence In Full Bloom Journal, write one way you can carry this peace into the day ahead.

Reflection: Ask yourself - How does calmness prepare me to show up as love in motion?

MIDDAY RITUAL – Open-heartedness and Optimism

As the day unfolds, let your heart open like a tender leaf leaning toward sunlight. Joy is the water that keeps self-love alive. In this moment, let yourself delight in something small, a smile exchanged, the warmth of tea between your hands, the sound of laughter. These gentle joys remind your spirit that growth is happening, right here, right now.

Mantra: I open my heart to sacred joy.

Action: Create a brief ritual of delight, a song, a slow walk, or a nourishing meal. Savor it fully. Let it be your reminder that joy is not a luxury, it's your light.

Reflection: Ask yourself - What does joy teach me about my worthiness to feel good, here, and now?

EVENING RITUAL – Manifestation

As dusk drapes softly across your evening, bring your awareness back to what is quietly unfolding within you. Every breath, every kind thought, every gentle act is proof that you are growing. Close your eyes and picture your spirit expanding, tender yet unstoppable, radiant yet grounded.

Mantra: I am growing in grace and strength.

Action: In your Confidence In Full Bloom Journal, write about one part of yourself that feels more open or alive than before. Offer gratitude for that unfolding.

Reflection: Ask yourself - How does acknowledging my quiet growth deepen my trust in the path ahead?

CLOSING THOUGHT:

Tonight, rest in the knowing that your self-love has begun to reach the surface. What was once hidden now shimmers with color and possibility. Trust this tender beginning, it is how every bloom learns to meet the sun.

DAY 8: ALLOWING SELF-LOVE TO GROW

"Growth is not a rush, it is the rhythm of love learning to breathe between rest and becoming."

Ohayou gozaimasu (Japanese), Extraordinary Bloomer. Today, your self-love begins to stretch beyond the tender beginnings you've nurtured. Think of it like sunlight meeting the first open leaves, gentle, certain, alive. Growth asks that you listen, not push; that you flow, not force. It is the quiet unfolding that happens when you give yourself what you need and trust that it's enough.

MORNING RITUAL – Balance and Love

Begin your morning with your Self-Love Bloom Essentials , sip your Restore Tea Blend, flow through your Release Yoga Sequence, and breathe in your Radiance Essential Oil Blend. Let these rituals draw you into balance. Growth cannot thrive in depletion; it requires nourishment, rest, and grace. When you meet yourself in the stillness, you fill your cup before you pour into others.

Mantra: I am nourished by balance and guided by love.

Action: Give yourself a slow, grounding moment this morning, a mindful stretch, a calm breakfast, or a few breaths of gratitude. Let it be enough.

Reflection: Ask yourself - How does beginning my day in balance shape the way I show myself love?

MIDDAY RITUAL – Open-heartedness and Optimism

As the day opens, so do you. Let your heart stretch toward connection, share warmth, offer kindness, or savor beauty in the smallest places. Growth is sustained by joy, and joy is amplified through giving and receiving light. When you share from a full spirit, optimism becomes your natural state.

Mantra: My love grows brighter when shared with others.

Action: Choose one Bloom Booster from your BYO or Appendix B:3b that brings you joy, perhaps a walk in sunlight, a moment of laughter, or sharing gratitude aloud.

Reflection: Ask yourself - How did opening my heart to joy expand my sense of peace and possibility today?

EVENING RITUAL – Manifestation

As the day fades, return to your center. Growth settles quietly at dusk, it roots deeper, unseen yet unstoppable. Let your breath slow. Reflect on how you nurtured your balance and shared your light. Self-love manifests through awareness; when you see your progress, you strengthen it.

Mantra: I manifest balance and peace through gentle growth.

Action: In your **Confidence in Full Bloom Journal**, write one way you grew in self-love today and one gentle intention for tomorrow's nourishment.

Reflection: Ask yourself - What did today teach me about growing without rushing?

CLOSING THOUGHT:

Tonight, rest knowing that your growth is steady, sacred, and yours alone. You are learning the art of balance, the grace of giving and receiving love in equal measure. Every act of care, every exhale of peace, is proof that you are already blooming.

DAY 9: HONORING YOUR BLOOM

"The moment you pause to see your own beauty, the garden within you exhales in gratitude."

Buenos días (Chilean), Ravishing Bloomer. . Today is about reverence, for your strength, your tenderness, your becoming. You have tended the soil of self-worth, watered the roots of self-efficacy, and nourished the petals of self-love. Now, like a flower turned toward morning light, you pause to honor your own bloom, not for perfection, but for presence. Honoring your growth is an act of grace. It's saying, *I have come this far, and I am still unfolding.*

MORNING RITUAL – Balance and Love

Begin your morning slowly. Sip your Restore Tea Blend and feel the warmth remind you of how often you've chosen to show up for yourself. Move through your Release Yoga Sequence, breathe in your Radiance Blend, and let gratitude rise like sunlight through leaves. This quiet noticing , this awareness , is the love that sustains you.

Mantra: I honor my growth and evolution.

Action: In your Confidence In Full Bloom Journal, write three moments in this journey where you surprised yourself , where love steadied you, courage guided you, or gentleness softened your way forward.

Reflection: Ask yourself - Which of these moments feel like sunlight I can still feel on my skin today?

MIDDAY RITUAL – Open-heartedness and Optimism

Let the afternoon be a gentle dance. Growth isn't always solemn , it's laughter, light, and the sacred joy of realizing how alive you've become. Step into that joy. Let your body remember it, let your spirit play.

Mantra: I open to sacred play and freedom.

Action: Do something playful , sway to music, walk barefoot in the grass, stretch beneath the sky, or smile at your reflection as if you were greeting a dear friend.

Reflection: Ask yourself - How did allowing play to enter my day lift my spirit and open my heart to more love?

EVENING RITUAL – Manifestation

As the evening settles, rest in the awareness of your fullness. You are both the seed and the bloom , still growing, still glowing. Envision what it means to live from this self-love every day. Tomorrow, you will celebrate your full bloom; tonight, you simply honor that it's already here.

Mantra: I am ready to live as love in bloom.

Action: In your **Confidence In Full Bloom Journal**, write one intention you will carry into tomorrow's celebration. Let it be something radiant and real , "I will walk in joy," "I will rest in peace," or "I will shine without apology."

Reflection: Ask yourself - How does recognizing my own wholeness prepare me to bloom even brighter?

CLOSING THOUGHT:

Tonight, let gratitude be your lullaby. You have tended your heart with patience, joy, and grace , and now, it blooms. Tomorrow, you will celebrate not just what you've done, but who you've become. Rest knowing: your love is already in full bloom.

DAY 10: CELEBRATING IN FULL BLOOM

"There comes a moment when the garden no longer asks for tending, only your presence, your joy, your awe."

Ekaro (Yoruba), Exquisite Bloomer. Today, we celebrate *you.* The fullness of your journey. The grace of your unfolding. The woman who has shown up, again and again, with courage, compassion, and care. You are standing in the season of your own bloom, where your self-worth, self-efficacy, and self-love intertwine like sunlight, roots, and rain. This is your harvest day, the moment to honor how beautifully you've grown.

MORNING RITUAL – Balance and Love

Begin softly. Sip your Restore Tea Blend and taste the warmth of your own becoming. Flow through your Release Yoga Sequence, breathing deeply as you remember all the times you chose yourself, quietly, steadily, faithfully. This morning is not about striving but integrating. You have gathered so much light; now let it settle into wholeness.

Mantra: I am balanced, loved, and whole.

Action: In your **Confidence In Full Bloom Journal**, write a love note to yourself. Begin with, *"Dear Me, I'm proud of you because..."* Let your words be honest and tender.

Reflection: Ask yourself - How does acknowledging my own devotion deepen my sense of balance and self-trust?

MIDDAY RITUAL – Open-heartedness and Optimism

Let the day feel expansive. Open the windows. Play music that moves you. Let joy be your prayer. Celebration need not be loud; it only needs to be *true*. Whether you share laughter with loved ones or savor solitude in sunlight, let your joy ripple outward.

Mantra: I open my heart to joy, gratitude, and celebration.

Action: Choose a simple act of celebration, walk among flowers, write a gratitude list, take yourself to lunch, or dance barefoot in your living room. Let it feel like *enough*.

Reflection: Ask yourself - What does celebration teach me about honoring my own becoming?

EVENING RITUAL – Manifestation

As night falls, close your eyes and breathe into the memory of these ten days, the soft starts, the small victories, the tender turning points. You have been cultivating more than habits; you have been shaping a way of being. Let this reflection become your map for what comes next.

Mantra: I manifest my purpose and live as love in bloom.

Action: In your Confidence In Full Bloom Journal, write three things you will continue to nurture, one for your body, one for your mind, and one for your spirit. Let them become your compass for the days ahead.

Reflection: Ask yourself - How does this moment of reflection help me trust that my self-love will keep unfolding long after today?

CLOSING THOUGHT:

Tonight, rest inside your own radiance. You have journeyed from seed to sunlight, from intention to embodiment. Your self-love is no longer an idea, it is alive, breathing through your choices, glowing through your presence.

Take one last sip of tea, one deep breath of gratitude, and remember: *You are not becoming the bloom. You are the bloom.*

PHASE 3 – SELF-LOVE: CLOSING SUMMARY

My dear Radiant Bloomer. You've completed the ten-day journey of *Self-Love*, a sacred season of remembering, returning, and rising into your own light. Over these days, you've tended the inner garden of your spirit, learning that love is not something you wait to receive, it's something you cultivate, day by day, breath by breath.

You began by planting seeds of gratitude and vision, seeing yourself with fresh eyes and daring to imagine your wholeness. You learned the quiet strength of commitment, the nourishment of gentleness, and the art of replenishment through presence and rest. You rooted into balance, opened to joy, and allowed your love to grow, stretch, and bloom in fullness. Each reflection, each ritual, each small act of devotion became proof that love has always been growing within you.

This phase followed the **BLOOM Bloomprint cadence:**

- **Morning – Balance and Love:** You began each day grounded in care, sipping your tea, breathing deeply, and tending to your body, mind, and spirit with gentleness.
- **Midday – Open-heartedness and Optimism:** You practiced connection and joy, expanding your heart through gratitude, play, and acts of kindness that kept your love alive and flowing.
- **Evening – Manifestation:** You closed each day with intention and reflection, honoring your growth and envisioning the radiant life that continues to unfold before you.

Your *Bloom At-Home Spiritual Wellness Practices* guided your evolution, mindful journaling, loving affirmations, heart-centered rituals, gentle movement, and daily gratitude. These practices became living prayers, grounding you in self-compassion, joy, and renewal.

- Through this journey, you've learned to:
- See yourself through the lens of grace and reverence.
- Balance giving and receiving love without guilt or depletion.
- Anchor joy and rest as acts of devotion.
- Trust that your wholeness is not something to earn, it is something to embody.

This phase has revealed that self-love is not a destination but a *daily dialogue* between your heart and your higher self. It is the rhythm of returning home, to your breath, your truth, and your boundless worthiness.

- Carry forward the rhythm of **BLOOM:**
- Begin with **Balance**, honoring your needs.
- Lead with **Love**, rooted in compassion.
- Stay **Open-hearted**, choosing joy and connection.
- Embody **Optimism**, trusting in your continued unfolding.
- **Manifest** your truth through daily intention and care.

You've now completed the third leg of your *Confidence In Full Bloom* journey, and what a beautiful becoming it's been. Take a deep, slow breath. Feel the warmth of your own radiance settling in your chest. You are not just blooming, you *are* the bloom, vibrant and whole.

When you're ready, complete your *Post-Blooming Self-Love Quick Assessment* to reflect on your growth and spiritual wellness.

Post – Blooming Self-Love Quick Assessment

Instructions: For each statement, rate yourself from **1 (Not at all true)** to **5 (Completely true).** Tally your score at the end and compare to Day 0.

Part 1: Quick Self-Check

		1-5
1	I prioritize time for activities that bring me joy.	
2	I allow myself to receive love from others.	
3	I nurture my body with food, movement, and rest.	
4	I forgive myself when I make mistakes.	
5	I offer love, compassion, and patience to myself regularly.	
6	I set boundaries to protect my energy and well-being.	
7	I speak to myself with kindness and encouragement.	
8	I celebrate my strengths and achievements without guilt.	
9	I accept myself fully, flaws and all.	
	Total	

Part 2: Blooming Reflections:

What shifted most for me over the last 10 days?

Which practice(s) felt the most empowering for me?

Part 3: My Victory Statement

In your journal, write a short declaration that celebrates your blooming.

Post Spiritual Wellness Check-in: Shade and name the pie.

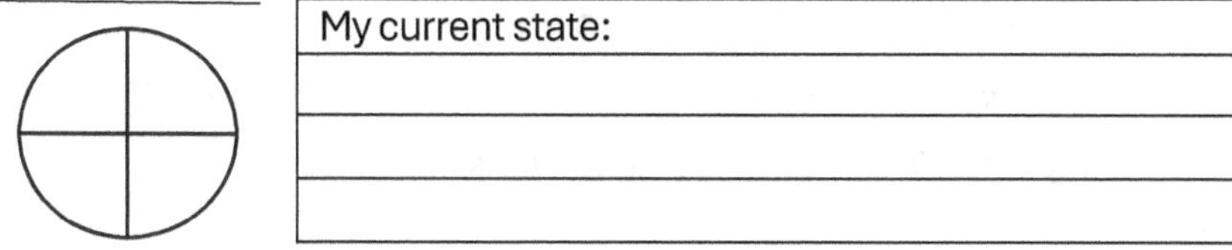

Confidence In Full Bloom Celebration: A Season of Returning to Love

Congratulations, Confident Bloomer. You've completed your *Confidence In Full Bloom* journey; a 30-day return to love, presence, and purpose. This isn't just the close of a chapter; it's a tea-worthy moment of reflection, celebration, and gratitude for how far you've come.

You have tended to your self-worth, cultivated self-efficacy, and blossomed in self-love. You've planted seeds of confidence, watered them with intention, and watched them take root in your daily life. And now, here you stand, radiant, rooted, and blooming.

To honor your growth, gather your favorite cup and steep a pot of your Restore Tea Blend. Make this a ceremony; a *Tea for One* (my go to) or *Tea for Three* celebration with your friends. Surround yourself with beauty: your Confidence in Full Bloom Journal, the plant you've nurtured along this journey, soft music, maybe even fresh flowers.

Then, choose one or more ways to celebrate your season of returning to love:

1. **Host a Blooming Tea Party.** Invite friends or family to sip tea, share stories, and speak words of affirmation to one another.
2. **Tend Your Plant.** The same one you've been growing these 30 days, repot it, water it, and place it in the sunlight as a living symbol of your self-love taking root.

3. **Write a Love Letter to Yourself.** Reflect on how you've changed, what you've reclaimed, and how you'll continue to honor your growth.
4. **Create a Gratitude Jar.** Fill it with moments, lessons, and wins from your journey.
5. **Celebrate Through Art.** Paint, dance, sing, or collage your transformation into something beautiful and lasting.
6. **Host a Personal Reflection Picnic.** Take your tea, your journal, and your plant outdoors. Let nature witness your joy.
7. **Light a Candle or Burn Incense.** Say aloud: "I am confident. I am worthy. I am in full bloom."
8. **Gift Yourself Rest.** Take a slow morning or a digital-free day to bask in the peace you've earned.

Whatever you choose, do it with presence and tenderness. Let your celebration mirror the woman you've become, soft yet strong, still yet expansive, blooming in her own rhythm.

Closing Thought:

This is your moment, your harvest, your bloom. You have returned to love, not as a visitor, but as its keeper. Breathe it in. Sip your tea slowly. And know, deep in your bones, that you are the garden and the gardener, forever growing toward the light.

Blooming Reflection: Returning to Love

> Let me tell you a story about a sunflower.
>
> She didn't bloom all at once. She rose slowly, seed, stem, then something brave and golden stretching toward the sun.
>
> She laughed with the wind, bowed to the rain, and kept her face turned toward the light, even when it hid behind the clouds.
>
> Like the others in the garden, she never realized how much good she was doing just by being herself.
>
> Her roots healed the weary soil beneath her. Her wide face fed the honeybees, the hummingbirds, and the redbirds that came seeking sweetness. Her broad leaves sheltered the small ones, orange and green geckos hiding from heat and harm.
>
> She didn't need to be a rose or a lily or anything more delicate than her own truth. Her gold was enough. Her purpose, whole.
>
> There were days she drooped under the weight of weather when her brightness felt spent. But love never left her. It waited, patient, constant, until she turned toward it again.
>
> That is the quiet miracle of this journey: to heal what holds you, to feed what needs you, to bloom without apology.
>
> Because when you return to love, daily, gently, confidently, intentionally...
>
> love returns to you multiplied.

Appendix

Here Is Your Garden's Tool Shed

This is your go-to corner for extras that will help your confidence and wellness journey thrive. Think of it as your personal toolshed, filled with practical resources, joyful practices, and inspiration to keep your garden growing long after your 30-day adventure.

Inside, you'll find:

- Appendix A: Tools List - A list of all the essentials and nice-to-have options that make your Bloom Practice come alive.
- Appendix B: Bloom At-Home Wellness Practices: Simple rituals and boosters you can use anytime to nurture your mind, body, and spirit.
- Appendix C: Life-Long Learning Resources: Books, guides, and ideas to feed your curiosity, creativity, and ongoing growth.
- Appendix D: References

Use this section like a garden shed: pick what you need, play with it, and let it help your inner garden flourish every day.

Appendix A:
Your Bloom Tools List

☐ Confidence In Full Bloom Journal *(optional enhancement)*

Your personal sanctuary in writing, a place to record your reflections, breakthroughs, and "aha" moments throughout this guide. It pairs perfectly with your *Confidence In Full Bloom* journey, helping you witness your own growth, one page at a time.

☐ My Life In Full Bloom Planner *(optional enhancement)*

For those who love structure and reflection, the *My Life In Full Bloom Planner* offers space to align your confidence practice with your daily life. Use it to track habits, set intentions, and celebrate your wins season by season.

☐ Favorite Pen or Pencil Set

Choose something that feels good in your hand and inspires you to linger on the page. A few colorful pens or pencils can bring lightness and creativity to your reflection time.

☐ Your Practice Nook

Designate a cozy space where you can focus and exhale. A sunny chair, a quiet corner, or a shady spot outdoors, all perfect choices. Over time, this becomes your sanctuary, a space that gently reminds your mind and body, *"This is where I return to myself."*

☐ Comfort + Wellness Essentials

Elevate your *Bloom-At-Home Wellness* rituals with a few nurturing companions:

- **Herbal teas and a tea diffuser** (a French press works beautifully), see Appendix B for seasonal recipes.
- **Essential and carrier oils** (Castor, Coconut, Jojoba)find blends in each phase to ground, energize, or uplift.
- **Smoothies or nourishing sips:** treat your body like the vessel of confidence it is. Recipes and guidance appear throughout the guide. *(Tip: Choose Certified Organic ingredients and products whenever possible.)*

☐ Openness, Curiosity, and Willingness to Grow

The most important tools aren't things you can buy; they're the qualities you bring to the process. Show up with openness, curiosity, and compassion. With these in hand, you're already preparing the soil for something beautiful to bloom: a confidence that feels rooted, radiant, and real.

Appendix B: Bloom At-Home Wellness

To grow confidence that lasts, you need more than motivation , you need nourishment. These **Bloom-At-Home Wellness practices** are your sunlight, rain, and rich soil , gentle supports that help your roots grow deeper as you strengthen your emotional, physical, and spiritual wellness.

Each phase of your journey focuses on one of these three wellness dimensions:

- **Emotional Wellness** helps you understand, express, and manage your feelings in ways that bring balance and resilience. It's learning to pause, name what you feel, and respond with compassion instead of criticism. Emotional wellness builds the foundation of self-worth , that quiet confidence that says, *"I am valuable, capable, and deserving of care."*
- **Physical Wellness** helps you reconnect to your body's natural rhythms. Through rest, nourishment, gentle movement, and mindful breathing, you learn to listen to your body's signals instead of pushing past them. Physical wellness is confidence in motion , a daily act of respect for the body that carries you.
- **Spiritual Wellness** centers your connection to meaning and presence , whatever that looks like for you. It's the reminder that you are part of something larger, that your life has purpose, and that peace is possible right where you are. Spiritual

wellness turns confidence into grace , calm, grounded, and luminous.

THE PRACTICE STRUCTURE

Each phase includes two kinds of wellness support designed to meet you exactly where you are:

1. Bloom Essentials

Your daily touchpoints , simple practices that blend seamlessly into everyday life. Think calming tea rituals, aromatherapy moments, mindful breathing, or a three-pose yoga flow that resets your energy. These are your daily anchors , small, steady acts of care that build confidence from the inside out.

2. Bloom Boosters

Optional enhancements that expand your wellness toolkit. These might include journaling prompts, mindful movies for reflection, basil-infused green smoothies, nature walks, or playlists for mood elevation. They're extra sunlight for the days you want to shine brighter.

You'll mix and match from these to create your own **Build-Your-Own (BYO) Bloom-At-Home Wellness Plan** , because your path is personal. There's no one right way to bloom. Trust your intuition. Listen to your body. Choose what feels nourishing and realistic for your lifestyle.

How to Use This Section

1. **Explore the options.** Skim through both lists in each phase , Essentials, and Boosters.
2. **Select what resonates.** Choose a few practices that fit your energy, space, and needs.
3. **Create your rhythm.** Use your BYO worksheet to build a weekly routine that feels supportive, not stressful.
4. **Engage consistently.** The more often you practice, the more you'll notice subtle shifts , calmer mornings, clearer thoughts, and a softer heart toward yourself.

Every small act of care is a seed of confidence. Every mindful choice helps your emotional, physical, and spiritual wellness flourish in harmony. Over time, those roots of wellness grow into the kind of confidence that doesn't shake when life does.

A GENTLE WORD OF CAUTION (Mmm-hmm)

These practices are here to **nurture your wellness**, not replace professional or medical care. Everyone's body, health history, and needs are unique. If you are pregnant, managing a chronic condition, or healing from illness or injury, modify or skip any practice that doesn't feel right for you.

Use your **Build-Your-Own Bloom-At-Home Wellness Plan worksheet** to select what supports your energy, your health, and your joy, so your mind, body, and spirit can flourish safely and beautifully.

Appendix B:1a - Bloom Essentials for Emotional Wellness

Your self-worth flourishes when you intentionally nurture your mind, body, and spirit. These Emotional Wellness staples are your daily anchors, simple, accessible practices you can return to again and again. They invite you to slow down, connect with your body, and remind yourself of your value.

Each day in this phase, you are encouraged to practice three times a day: morning, midday, and bedtime, with these rituals: sipping a grounding tea, moving through a short yoga sequence, and breathing in uplifting aromatherapy. These consistent acts of care help you feel steady, radiant, and aligned with your worth.

REVITALIZE - HERBAL TEA BLEND

This gentle blend is designed to ground, calm, and uplift your spirit while supporting emotional balance.

Ingredients (per cup):

- ¼ tsp Holy Basil (Tulsi) – reduces stress, fosters clarity
- ¼ tsp Peppermint – refreshes and energizes the mind
- ¼ tsp Lemon Balm – relieves tension, promotes peace
- ½ tsp Chamomile – calms, soothes the nervous system (at bedtime only to relax.)

Instructions:

- Boil 1 cup of water and allow it to cool slightly (ideal temp: 190–200°F).
- Place herbs in a tea infuser, teapot, or directly into a mug.

- Pour the hot water over the herbs and cover to steep for 5–7 minutes. Covering keeps the beneficial oils in.
- Strain if needed. Sip slowly, breathing deeply between sips.

Tip: Prepare a larger batch (2–3 cups) in the morning and sip throughout the day.

RENEW - YOGA SEQUENCE

Yoga grounds you in presence and connects you to your inner strength. Choose the version that works best for your body, traditional standing poses, or seated adaptations, or mix and match as you go.

Traditional

1. **Mountain Pose:** (Tadasana):Stand tall with feet hip-width apart, grounding evenly through both feet. Lengthen your spine, relax your shoulders, arms resting by your sides. Feel your dignity and presence rise with each inhale.

2. **Warrior II:** (Virabhadrasana II):Step one foot back 3–4 feet, front knee bent over ankle, back leg strong. Extend arms parallel to the floor, gaze over front fingertips. Root through your feet and expand through your chest, radiating strength and focus.

3. **Tree Pose:** (Vrksasana**):**Shift weight onto one foot, placing the sole of the other foot on your ankle, calf, or thigh (avoid the knee). Press palms together at your heart or extend arms overhead. Root down while lifting up, embodying stability and grace.

Seated

1. **Seated Mountain:**
   Sit near the edge of a sturdy chair, feet flat on the ground. Press down through your sit bones, lengthen your spine, and rest your hands on your thighs or at your sides. Inhale, imagining yourself grounded yet lifted.

2. **Seated Warrior II:**
   Sit sideways on the chair, legs open in a lunge-like position if space allows. Extend arms outward, gaze over your front fingertips. Feel strength and openness across your chest.

3. **Seated Tree**:
   Sit tall, feet grounded. Cross one ankle over the opposite shin or place foot gently along the calf. Bring palms together at your chest or raise arms overhead. Root down through your sit bones, lifting through your crown.

Practice whichever sequence feels supportive, holding each pose for 3–5 breaths before moving to the next.

REFRESH – AROMATHERAPY ESSENTIAL OILS BLEND

Scent is a powerful ally in emotional wellness. This blend invites calm, balance, and confidence into your day.

Ingredients:

- 2 tablespoons carrier oil (sweet almond, jojoba, or coconut oil)
- 3 drops lavender essential oil (calming, grounding)
- 2 drops bergamot essential oil (uplifting, confidence-enhancing)
- 1 drop patchouli essential oil (stability, self-acceptance)

Instructions:

- **Massage Oil**: Combine carrier oil and essential oils in a glass bottle. Gently shake. Massage onto chest, shoulders, or hands while repeating a loving affirmation, such as: *"I am worthy of love and joy."*
- **Diffuser**: Add 5–6 drops of the blend (without carrier oil) to a diffuser to fill your space with warmth and positivity.
- **Pocket Inhaler**: Place a cotton ball in a small glass jar or clean spice bottle. Add just the essential oils (without carrier oil). Inhale deeply throughout the day when you need grounding or a boost of confidence. Replace cotton every 2–3 days.

Daily Integration

Morning, midday, and bedtime, return to your three essentials: sip your herbal tea with presence, move through your yoga sequence, and invite in supportive aromas. Over time, these repeated actions create a rhythm that reminds you: *You are rooted. You are radiant. You are worthy.*

Appendix B:1b - Bloom Boosters for Emotional Wellness

Choose and try out the Bloom Boosters that speak to you. You can also include your own.

Mindfulness & Grounding: Start each practice by taking 2–3 deep breaths, feeling your feet on the floor, and noticing sensations in your body. This simple act centers your attention, calms your nervous system, and prepares your mind and heart to fully engage in any activity.

Gratitude Mirror Work: Sit in front of a mirror, make eye contact with yourself, and write down three things you love about who you are becoming. Read them aloud slowly and kindly. This ritual reframes inner dialogue and anchors your sense of worth. Or, stand before a mirror and say one loving affirmation, such as: "I am worthy of love exactly as I am." Repeat 3 times slowly and gently. This strengthens confidence and transforms limiting beliefs.

Gratitude Letter to Self: Write a short note of gratitude addressed to yourself. Acknowledge your strengths, efforts, and resilience. Seal it and open it whenever you need a reminder of your worth. This reinforces self-recognition and appreciation.

Tapping (EFT – Emotional Freedom Technique): Use gentle tapping on energy points: side of hand, eyebrow, side of eye, under eye, under nose, chin, collarbone, under arm, and top of head, while focusing on a challenge, worry, or limiting belief. Say: "I am capable." This releases tension, frees emotional blocks, and boosts self-belief.

Resilience Reset Reflection: Recall a past setback where you bounced back. Journal what helped you recover and what it taught you about your strength. This reinforces emotional resilience.

Digital Garden Reset: Spend an hour decluttering your digital space, delete old emails, organize your desktop, and unsubscribe from draining content. Imagine weeding your mental garden to make room for self-worth and clarity to flourish.

Bloom Cinema Reflection: Choose films that celebrate courage, resilience, or self-love, such as *Hidden Figures, Eat Pray Love, Wild,* or *The Color Purple.* After watching, journal: "What did this story teach me about believing in myself, and where do I see my own worth reflected in it?" This combines inspiration, reflection, and emotional growth.

Bloom Music: Let music become your companion for healing. Create playlists that lift your spirit, calm your mind, or help you process emotions. Whether it's singing, playing an instrument, or simply listening, sound can shift your mood and open new doors of expression.

Art and Drawing: Give your feelings a canvas. Drawing, painting, coloring, or even doodling allows emotions to flow in nonverbal ways, creating clarity and release. This is not about being an artist; it's about using color and form to reflect your inner landscape.

Appendix B:2a - Bloom Essentials for Self-Efficacy

Self-efficacy is about trusting your ability to take action, make choices, and follow through on your goals. To support this, these physical wellness practices energize your body, sharpen your focus, and remind you of your strength. Each time you sip your tea, move through your yoga poses, or breathe in your aromatherapy blend, you are building momentum and reinforcing the truth that you can grow, thrive, and succeed.

When practiced morning, midday, and bedtime, these simple rituals become your anchors. They help you center yourself, claim your power, and approach your day with clarity, courage, and confidence.

RECHARGE - HERBAL TEA BLEND

This herbal blend is crafted to awaken energy, sharpen focus, and strengthen resilience.

Ingredients:

- ½ teaspoon green tea
- ¼ teaspoon peppermint
- ¼ teaspoon ginger
- ¼ teaspoon lemon peel

Instructions:

- Boil 1 cup of water and allow it to cool slightly (ideal temp: 190–200°F).
- Place herbs in a tea infuser, teapot, or directly into a mug.

- Pour the hot water over the herbs and cover to steep for 5–7 minutes. Covering keeps the beneficial oils in.
- Strain if needed. Sip slowly, breathing deeply between sips.

In the morning, enjoy this tea as a way to set intention for the day. Midday, use it to re-energize and refocus. In the evening, take a gentler sip, reflecting on your wins, no matter how small. Each cup becomes a reminder that your body and mind are capable, focused, and strong.

RISE – YOGA SEQUENCE

Yoga helps you embody focus, strength, and perseverance. The poses below are presented in both traditional standing forms and seated modifications, so you can choose what works best for your body. Repeat the sequence morning, midday, and bedtime, adjusting the intensity as needed.

Traditional Sequence - Energy

1. **Warrior I:** (Virabhadrasana I): Step one foot back about three to four feet. Bend the front knee directly over the ankle, keeping the back leg long and grounded. Lift both arms overhead, palms facing each other. Gaze forward or slightly upward. Root firmly into the earth through your feet while lifting your chest with confidence.

2. **Chair Pose:** (Utkatasana): Stand with feet hip-width apart. Bend your knees as if lowering into an invisible chair, keeping the weight in your heels and the knees behind your toes. Lift your arms overhead, chest open, core engaged. Hold and breathe steadily, feeling your strength build.

3. **Plank Pose:** (Phalakasana): Begin on hands and toes, aligning shoulders directly over wrists. Keep your body in a straight line from head to heels. Engage your core and thighs, pressing strongly through your hands. Hold as long as steady breath allows, cultivating resilience and focus.

Seated Sequence

1. **Warrior I**: Sit tall near the edge of a chair. Extend one leg slightly forward and the other back if space allows or keep both feet firmly on the floor. Lift your arms overhead, palms together or shoulder-width apart, and lift your chest while grounding through your sit bones.

2. **Chair Pose:** Sit tall with feet flat on the floor. Hinge slightly forward from the hips, reaching arms overhead. Press firmly into your feet and draw your core in, imagining the engagement of your thighs and lower body as though standing in the traditional pose.

3. **Mini Plank**: Sit near the edge of a sturdy chair. Place your hands firmly on the seat or edge beside your hips. Step your feet slightly forward, straightening your legs comfortably. Press into your hands, lift your chest, and engage your core, feeling the activation of a plank. Hold for a few breaths, keeping shoulders relaxed. Do not do this on a slippery floor.

RESILIENT – ESSENTIAL OIL BLEND AROMATHERAPY

Scent is a powerful trigger for focus, clarity, and confidence. This blend is designed to awaken your energy, sharpen your mind, and root you in resilience.

Ingredients:

- 2 tablespoons carrier oil such as jojoba, sweet almond, or coconut oil
- 3 drops lemon essential oil for clarity and motivation
- 2 drops rosemary essential oil for focus and mental sharpness
- 1 drop ginger essential oil for energy and confidence.

Instructions:

- **Massage:** Blend oils together in a small glass bottle. Apply a few drops to your chest, shoulders, or hands while repeating an empowering affirmation such as "I am capable and strong."

- **Diffuser**: Add four to six drops of the essential oils (without the carrier oil) to a diffuser and allow the scent to fill your space, creating an atmosphere of clarity and focus.

- **Inhaler:** Place a cotton ball in a small glass or medicine bottle. Drop the essential oils directly onto the cotton ball, then close with a lid when not in use to preserve potency. Inhale as needed throughout the day, especially before tackling a challenge or setting a new goal. Replace the cotton ball every two to three days.

Always perform a small patch test before applying oils to the skin to ensure there is no sensitivity.

Appendix B:2b - Bloom Boosters for Physical Wellness

Your body is your foundation for strength, vitality, and confidence. These practices go beyond the basics to restore energy, encourage resilience, and remind you that caring for your body is an act of empowerment. Try one or two daily as add-ons to your wellness staples. Each practice strengthens your physical well-being while also nurturing your self-trust and self-efficacy.

EMPOWERING MOVEMENT & CARE

Hydrotherapy Reset

Take a refreshing shower or alternate warm and cool water over your body. Breathe deeply as the water flows and silently affirm, "I wash away doubt, I awaken strength." This practice stimulates circulation, clears heaviness, and recharges your energy.

Dry Brushing Ritual

Before bathing, use a natural-bristle brush on dry skin. Start at your feet and brush upward toward your heart with long, gentle strokes. Repeat on arms from hands to shoulders. This simple ritual boosts circulation, exfoliates the skin, and helps your body feel renewed.

Blooming Herbal Bath or Foot Soak

Combine rose petals, lavender, and a pinch of sea salt in warm water. Soak your body or feet while repeating, "My body is worthy of rest and care." As you relax, imagine tension melting away and your skin absorbing nourishment and vitality.

Self-Massage with Bloom Oil

Choose a nourishing oil such as almond, coconut, or jojoba and add a drop of jasmine or ylang-ylang essential oil. Massage into arms, shoulders, and chest with slow, mindful strokes. Thank your body for its strength and capability with every touch.

Heart-Centered Self-Massage

Focus gently on the chest and heart space. Use slow circular motions while silently repeating, "I honor my body's strength and resilience." This touch anchors self-efficacy and self-appreciation in the body.

Walking Practice

Take a 10–20 minute walk outdoors if possible. With each step, notice the rhythm of your feet and the movement of your breath. Walk with purpose, repeating a phrase like, "I move forward with strength." Walking boosts circulation, clears the mind, and connects you with your inner drive.

Dance for Joy

Put on music that uplifts you and move freely, whether for two minutes or twenty. Let your body express energy and emotion without worrying about steps or form. Dancing increases circulation, raises mood, and awakens confidence through joyful movement.

Restorative Sleep and Rest Ritual

Make your sleep environment calm and welcoming. Dim lights an hour before bed, silence unnecessary notifications, and sip a calming herbal tea. Before lying down, place a hand over your heart and affirm, "I allow my body to restore itself." Deep, regular rest strengthens resilience and restores energy for the day ahead.

Hydration with Clean Water:

Drink fresh, clean water throughout the day. Aim for at least six to eight cups, adjusting to your body's needs. Choose filtered or spring water when possible, minimizing exposure to PFAS and other contaminants. Each glass of water is a reset, supporting energy, focus, and clarity.

PFAS Purge:

Gradually reduce products that may contain PFAS (per- and polyfluoroalkyl substances), which are often found in nonstick cookware, fast-food wrappers, and some cosmetics. Replace nonstick pans with stainless steel or cast iron, choose uncoated paper for food storage, and check labels for "fluoro" ingredients. Each small swap supports your body's long-term health and helps reduce toxic load.

EMPOWERING SMOOTHIES – FUEL YOUR CONFIDENCE

Red Power Smoothie

- ½ cup strawberries
- ½ cup raspberries
- ½ fresh beet
- 4–5 fresh basil or mint leaves
- 5–6 red grapes
- 1 teaspoon chia seeds
- 1 cup cold water or coconut water

Blend until smooth. Sip mindfully, imagining each sip fueling your body with courage and vitality.

Green Energy Glow Smoothie

- 1 cup spinach
- 1 banana
- ½ cucumber
- ½ cup pineapple
- 4–5 basil leaves
- 1 cup coconut water

Blend and enjoy slowly. Let the refreshing taste remind you of the nourishment and energy you're giving your body to take bold action.

These are just some of the physical wellness bloom boosters available to you. If you have time, consider researching a few additional practices that you find engaging and add them to your BYO Bloom At-Home Wellness Plan.

A GENTLE WORD OF CAUTION: Yes again.

Please remember that these practices are here to inform you of methods to nurture your wellness, not replace medical treatment. Your body, health history, and circumstances are unique. If you are pregnant, managing diabetes, have heart disease, or any other medical condition, some of these practices may need modification.

Use your (BYO) Bloom At-Home Wellness Plan worksheet. To curate your own garden: you still get all the nourishment, sunlight, and growth, but in a way, that's perfectly suited to you.

Appendix B: 3a - Bloom Essentials for Spiritual Wellness

Self-love is about embracing all of who you are, nurturing your spirit, and celebrating your unique journey. These practices engage your mind, body, and spirit to open your heart, cultivate joy, and honor your needs. By practicing these rituals regularly, you build a foundation of love, acceptance, and inner harmony that radiates into every area of your life. Begin each session with a brief grounding: feel your feet on the floor, notice your body, and take three to five slow breaths to center yourself.

RESTORE – HERBAL TEA BLEND

This tea blend soothes the mind, comforts the spirit, and opens the heart, creating a mindful pause in your day. Each sip encourages reflection, presence, and gratitude.

Ingredients

- ½ tsp Hibiscus
- ½ tsp Rose Petals
- ¼ tsp Lemon Balm
- ¼ tsp Chamomile (add for relaxation)

Instructions:

- Boil 1 cup of water and allow it to cool slightly (ideal temp: 190–200°F).
- Place herbs in a tea infuser, teapot, or directly into a mug.
- Pour the hot water over the herbs and cover. Steep for 5–7 minutes. Covering keeps the beneficial oils in.
- Strain if needed. Sip slowly, breathing deeply between sips.

RELEASE - YOGA SEQUENCE

Traditional Yoga Poses:

- **Camel Pose** – Kneel with knees hip-width apart. Place your hands on your lower back or heels. Lift your chest and gently arch back, keeping your neck long. Breathe deeply into your heart space, expanding openness and courage.

- **Bound Angle Pose** – Sit on the floor, bring the soles of your feet together, and allow your knees to fall open. Hold your feet or ankles. Sit tall and soften your shoulders. Breathe into your hips and heart, cultivating grounded compassion.

- **Supported Child's Pose** – Kneel on the floor, bring your big toes together, and separate your knees comfortably. Fold forward, resting your chest and head on the mat. Extend arms forward or alongside the body. Breathe deeply and allow surrender, self-compassion, and calm to fill your awareness.

Seated Yoga Modifications:

- **Camel Pose**: Sit tall on a chair, your feet flat. Place your hands on the seat or hips and gently lift the heart upward, opening the chest. Inhale to expand, exhale to soften.

- **Bound Angle Pose**: Sit in a chair, bring the soles of your feet together so the knees open outward comfortably. Place your hands on your thighs and gently press knees downward with each exhale. Maintain a tall spine and feel the heart space expand.

- **Supported Child's Pose**: Sit in a chair with feet flat on the floor. Fold gently forward over your thighs, resting your arms on your legs or a cushion on your lap. Focus on your breath and allow the body to relax into comfort and self-kindness.

RADIANCE – ESSENTIAL OIL BLEND

Aromatherapy stimulates the senses and encourages mindfulness, emotional balance, and spiritual alignment. These practices can be used at any time of day to cultivate presence, calm, and self-compassion.

Self-Love : Heart-Opening Oil

Ingredients:

- 2 tablespoons of carrier oil such as sweet almond, jojoba, or coconut oil.
- 3 drops of rose essential oil for love and emotional balance.
- 2 drops of orange essential oil for joy and optimism.
- 1 drop of frankincense essential oil for grounding and presence.

Instructions:

- **Massage**: Blend the carrier and essential oils in a small glass bottle. Apply gently to chest, shoulders, or hands while silently or aloud repeating a loving affirmation such as "I am worthy of love and joy." Focus on inhaling deeply with each movement, letting the scent anchor your awareness in self-love.

- **Diffuser**: Add three to five drops to a diffuser. Allow the fragrance to fill your space, creating a calming, heart-centered environment. Breathe slowly and mindfully.
- **Inhaler:** Place a cotton ball in a small glass or spice bottle. Add the essential oil drops directly to the cotton ball. Seal the bottle and inhale as needed throughout the day. Replace the cotton ball every two to three days for potency.

Patch Test Reminder – Always test a small amount on your skin to check for sensitivity before regular use.

Daily Routine:

Integrate these practices three times daily. Use them in the morning to center yourself and set intentions, at midday to reconnect with your heart and energy, and at bedtime to reflect, release, and nurture your inner self. Over time, these rituals create a reliable rhythm that strengthens spiritual wellness and deepens your experience of self-love.

Appendix B: 3b - Bloom Boosters for Spiritual Wellness

Your spiritual wellness is the inner garden where self-love grows. These Bloom Boosters are optional yet powerful practices that support your connection to yourself, your heart, and the world around you. They cultivate presence, joy, and compassion while enhancing your daily BLOOM practices. Use one or several each day, morning, midday, or evening, and create a rhythm that nourishes your spirit.

Loving-Kindness Meditation: Sit quietly with your back straight and one hand on your heart. Repeat silently: "May I be happy. May I be healthy. May I be loved. May I live with ease."

After several rounds for yourself, extend these wishes to a loved one, a neutral person, and finally to the world. Visualize warmth radiating from your heart with each breath. Notice the sense of connection and compassion expanding outward. Spend 5–10 minutes for a full practice.

Candle of Compassion Ritual: Light a candle and place it near a small flower or plant. Close your eyes and whisper three loving affirmations into the flame. Sit quietly for several minutes, imagining the light radiating from your heart outward, filling your space and body with kindness. Let this ritual anchor presence, intention, and gentle self-care.

Forest Bathing or Nature Savoring: Step outside and spend time mindfully observing the natural world. Notice colors, textures, scents, and sounds. Take slow, deep breaths, and fully absorb each moment. Feel your body grounded to the earth, your heart connected to life, and your mind calm. Even five to ten minutes can restore balance, belonging, and joy.

Box Breathing for Heartful Presence: Sit comfortably with your back straight. Inhale through your nose for four counts, hold for four, exhale through your mouth for four, and hold for four. Repeat this cycle four to six times. As you breathe, visualize energy moving through your heart, opening it to self-love and calm awareness. This practice can center you anytime you feel scattered or stressed.

Bloom Music Ritual: Choose music that makes you feel radiant, alive, and connected. Close your eyes and ask: What does this music awaken in me? Move, sway, or simply breathe in rhythm with the sound. Allow the music to deepen your awareness of self-worth, uplift your mood, and nourish your spirit.

Savoring Ritual: Select a small sensory pleasure: a cup of tea, a piece of chocolate, a few moments of sunlight on your skin, or a gentle touch. Slow down and notice every detail, letting gratitude fill your awareness. Use this ritual to heighten appreciation, presence, and connection to life's simple joys.

Heart-Centered Affirmation Breath: Place your hands over your heart. Inhale deeply, imagining love flowing inward. Exhale, imagining love radiating outward. Repeat five to seven times while pairing each breath with an affirmation such as: "I am love. I deserve joy. I give kindness." This practice strengthens self-compassion and spiritual alignment.

Gratitude Practice: Take a few minutes to reflect on three things you are grateful for today. Write them down or simply hold them in your mind. Feel how the warmth of gratitude expands through your body and into your interactions. Gratitude supports spiritual wellness by anchoring you in the abundance of your life.

Vagus Nerve Connection – Intentional Connection: Engage in gentle, mindful interaction with another person to stimulate the vagus nerve and release oxytocin, supporting calm, trust, and openness. You might hold a loved one's hand, offer a heartfelt hug, or maintain eye contact while speaking kindly and intentionally. As you connect, focus on deep, slow breathing together, noticing warmth, presence, and mutual care. This practice helps regulate your nervous system, calm the mind, and open the heart, creating a foundation for self-love and deeper connection.

Animal or Pet Therapy : Spend intentional time with an animal (a cat, dog, bird, or whatever you feel drawn to). Observe their presence, breathe alongside them, and connect with their unconditional energy. Even a few minutes of this interaction can increase oxytocin, lower stress, and remind you of the simple joy of being present.

These Bloom Boosters are designed to complement your daily Bloom Essentials. Choose practices that resonate with you each day and allow your spiritual wellness to deepen naturally. Remember that self-love is cultivated and nurtured, not earned, and these rituals are a way to honor and expand your connection to yourself.

Appendix C: Life-Long Bloom Resources

Here is a list of classes I've taken that you might find helpful.

Massive Open Online Courses (MOOCs)

1. **Inspirational Leadership: Leading with Sense** (Case Western Reserve University) A multi-course specialization that strengthens confidence through enhanced self-awareness, communication, and emotionally intelligent leadership. Ideal for cultivating inner clarity and resilience in leadership roles. Case Western Reserve University

2. **Workplace Well-being: How to Build Confidence and Manage Stress** (LTU) Learn practical strategies to manage workplace stress, build self-esteem, and advocate for your value at work, perfect for reinforcing self-efficacy in daily life. ltu.se

3. **Self-Esteem & Confidence Courses** (Coursera offerings) A broad catalog of courses on cultivating positive mindset, building self-worth, and assertiveness, from reputable institutions like UPenn and University of Colorado. Coursera

TED Talks

1. **Cultivating Unconditional Self-Worth** , Adia Gooden- Explores how embracing yourself beyond perfection allows for freedom, joy, and profound belonging. TED

2. **The Skill of Self-Confidence** , Dr. Ivan Joseph: This talk breaks down confidence as a learnable skill, emphasizing practice, authenticity, and daily self-affirmation. My Mooc

3. **How Do You Find Self-Worth?** Dr. Lisa Strohman (TEDx) A thoughtful exploration of what it means to truly value yourself beyond external validation. TED

MasterClass Classes

1. **How to Build Self-Worth**:

   Offers tools for cultivating enduring self-worth by deepening emotional stability, setting boundaries, and recognizing your inherent value. MasterClass

2. **How to Be More Confident**

   Breaks down confidence in practical terms, embracing your strengths and accepting your imperfections with grace. MasterClass

3. **How to Stop Comparing Yourself to Others**

   Teaches how to diminish the harmful habit of comparison and instead root yourself in self-appreciation and authentic self-expression. MasterClass

Appendix D: References

American City Business Journals. (2025). *Women in the workforce: Mid-year survey*. Bizwomen.

Forbes Media. (2025). *Women's job security and the impact of DEI cuts. Forbes.*

Gallup. (2025). *State of global well-being report*. Gallup, Inc.

Gallup & Walton Family Foundation. (2023). *Gen Z and STEM interest survey*. Gallup, Inc.

Harvard Business Review. (2023). *The sponsor effect: Why sponsorship matters for women*. Harvard Business Publishing.

HP Inc. (2024). *Future ready workplace survey*. HP Development Company, L.P.

Motley Fool. (2025). *Women and financial confidence report*. The Motley Fool.

National Institutes of Health. (2024). *Gender equity in leadership and sponsorship studies*. U.S. Department of Health and Human Services.

World Economic Forum. (2025). *Global gender gap report 2025*. World Economic Forum.

A Year of Returning to Love

If you've made it this far, take a deep breath and smile; you've already begun. You've tended to your confidence, rediscovered parts of yourself, and maybe even felt your heart soften in new ways.

But this is just the beginning.

In Full Bloom is more than a collection of books; it's a full-circle experience in self-reclamation and personal growth. Each guide in the ***"Returning to Love" In Full Bloom*** series is a season of growth for your inner garden: four sacred journeys designed to help you heal, trust, and live with your heart wide open again. You can begin any time because there's no wrong moment to return to love.

The Returning to Love series:

Confidence In Full Bloom – Available now

A 30-Day Guide to Growing Unshakable Confidence in Uncertain Times. For the woman ready to believe in her own voice again, to rebuild trust in her abilities, honor her worth, and move forward with clarity and grace.

Grace In Full Bloom - to be released 1-15-2026

A Gentle 30-Day Guide to Forgiveness. A soft space for release and renewal. Learn to let go of resentment, invite in compassion, and allow grace to mend what pain once divided.

Purpose In Full Bloom - to be released 2-15-2026

A 30-Day Guide to Living With Clarity and Intention. A soulful roadmap back to what truly matters. You'll rediscover your "why," realign your energy with your values, and begin leading your life with meaning and conviction.

Joy In Full Bloom - to be released 3-15-2026

A 30-Day Guide to Cultivating Lightness and Everyday Delight.

A radiant closing chapter that invites laughter, gratitude, and ease back into your days. You'll learn to savor life's beauty; both the simple and the spectacular and live from a place of joy.

ENHANCE YOUR JOURNEY

Your *Returning to Love* year can be enriched with a few companions designed to help your growth unfold with rhythm and intention:

☐ **The "My Life In Full Bloom" Planner** – A yearlong companion that bridges your guides with real life. Use it to plan, reflect, and celebrate your progress through each season of returning to love.

☐ **In Full Bloom Journals for each guide** – Safe spaces for your private reflections, dreams, and discoveries. Each journal complements its matching guide, helping you deepen your experience through writing, ritual, and self-expression.

You can move through these four guides across a year or take them whenever your soul calls for renewal. Some begin with *Confidence,* others with *Grace.* What matters most is that you begin.

Each *In Full Bloom* journey is a return, to wholeness, to self-trust, to peace, and ultimately, to love.

So, whenever you're ready, your garden awaits.

Coming Soon - A Year of *Becoming*

Love awakens you. But *becoming* is where you rise.

Once you've returned to love, within yourself, your story, and your life; it's time to stretch, to grow, and to step fully into who you're meant to be. *In Full Bloom's* **Year of Becoming** collection will guide you through the next chapter: one of courage, creativity, and conscious expansion.

These journeys are about embodiment, the beautiful, sometimes messy process of living what you've learned. They'll help you root confidence deeper, speak your truth louder, and show up for your dreams without apology.

THE BECOMING COLLECTION:

Boundaries In Full Bloom - to be released 6-15-2026

A 30-Day Guide to Saying No Without Guilt and Yes to Yourself

For the woman ready to stop people-pleasing and start honoring her peace. Learn how to set boundaries that protect your energy and reflect your worth.

Healing In Full Bloom - to be released 7-15-2026

A 30-Day Guide to Restoring Your Mind, Body, and Spirit. A gentle invitation to tend to your inner wounds, release survival mode, and reintroduce your body to rest and safety.

Authenticity In Full Bloom to be released 8-15-2026

A 30-Day Guide to Living True to Yourself. For those ready to shed old expectations and live from truth. Reconnect with your inner compass and rediscover the freedom of being fully, unapologetically you.

Resilience In Full Bloom to be released 9-15-2026

A 30-Day Guide to Rising Stronger Than Before. A transformative journey into strength, faith, and flexibility. You'll learn to bend without breaking and thrive through change with grace and power.

About The Author

A Personal Reflection

For me, Confidence In Full Bloom isn't just a book; it's a lifeline, a friend, and a quiet whisper that says, "Yes. You can." Because I've been there too.

Researching and writing these guides changed me. It reminded me of something I tell my students and clients all the time: We can do anything we are willing to learn how to do.

Confidence isn't something you're born with. It's something you cultivate, season by season, choice by choice, moment by moment. In a perfect world, we wouldn't need to learn it at all. We'd come into the world surrounded by people who know how to love us and who teach us how to love ourselves. But many of us didn't get enough of that because some of our folks simply couldn't give what they never received. So, we learn. We teach ourselves. And that's okay, because this kind of confidence, the kind we build with intention and tenderness, is the kind that lasts.

This is what the In Full Bloom collection is all about. Each guide is part of a seasonal journey, this year it's a full year of Returning to Love through confidence, grace, purpose, and joy. Together, these guides help you move through your personal seasons of growth, learning to trust yourself again, to forgive, to realign with purpose, and to rediscover joy in your everyday life.

I know how hard it can be out there. How easy it is to feel small, unseen, or disconnected while the world strolls by. But here's what I've learned, and maybe you have too:

We can't change the world until we learn to anchor ourselves.

We can't influence much until we can influence our own thoughts, choices, and energy.

That's where our real power begins.

Learning to hold your head high isn't arrogance. It's sacred witnessing.

It's self-love.

It's spiritual acknowledgment.

It's necessary.

It's the moment you say, "I see me. I see my growth. I see my light. I matter."

If you are wondering why I wrote this book, I wrote the book I needed, a guide that's practical but soulful, structured but full of heart, designed not to preach from the podium but to walk beside you and me through our own blooming. My hope is that it helps you recognize and stack your wins, quiet or bold, overdue, or brand new. Because they matter. You matter.

And remember this:

We're not throwing in the towel.

Not here. Not now. Not ever.

We're blooming forward, together.

Biography : Stacey Y. Clark

Stacey Y. Clark, M.Ed., is an educator, coach, and wellness guide on a mission to help women live deeply rooted, joyfully expressed lives, no matter where they are living.

With experience in education, instructional design, communications, technology, and holistic wellness, and a whole lot more, she designs transformational experiences that blend reflection, creativity, and soul work.

She is the author of the In Full Bloom Guides, the *Manifesting Wellness* series, and the *Kissing in the Kitchen* "Movie Foodie" activity and cookbook series (currently being reimagined). Her work helps women reclaim their voice, power, and purpose, one page, one practice, and one adventure at a time. When she isn't writing, you'll find Stacey gardening, running workshops, exploring new cultures and places, inventing stuff, delighting in art, taking tea, or savoring good food and great conversations.

Let's Connect

If this journey has stirred something in you, and you want to hear more from me, I'd love to stay in touch. Visit SYMOORE Publishing at www.symoorepub.com and join the **Blooming By Nature** Facebook group. And follow @symoorepub on Instagram. Your next bloom is right at your fingertips.

A Note of Gratitude

There are literally millions of book out there for you to choose from, but for some reason, you chose this one. Thank you for saying yes to this journey, and to yourself. For picking up this guide, for making space to reflect, and for daring to honor the voice inside you've so often downplayed.

Your presence in these pages is proof that growth is possible even after long winters. That acknowledgment is the sacred work of healing. Blooming isn't always loud, but it is always powerful.

Every reflection, every pause for breath, every sacred "yes" you whispered back to your soul, it matters. You matter.

Keep tending to your truth. Keep claiming your crown. And never forget, you are the garden and the gardener, the seed, and the sunshine. You are everything!

With deep gratitude and faith in your blossoming,

xoxo

Stacey

www.ingramcontent.com/pod-product-compliance
Lightning Source LLC
LaVergne TN
LVHW010657110826
845149LV00014B/3131

9781961228078